Janiger, Oscar.

A different kind of
healing.

A Different Kind of Healing

A DIFFERENT KIND OF HEALING

Doctors Speak Candidly
About Their Successes with
Alternative Medicine

OSCAR JANIGER, M.D.,
AND PHILIP GOLDBERG

A Jeremy P. Tarcher / Putnam Book
Published by G. P. Putnam's Sons • New York

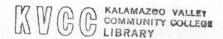

FEB 17 1994

A Jeremy P. Tarcher/Putnam Book
Published by G. P. Putnam's Sons
Publishers Since 1838
200 Madison Avenue
New York, NY 10016

Copyright © 1993 by Philip Goldberg and Oscar Janiger
All rights reserved. This book, or parts thereof,
may not be reproduced in any form without permission.
Requests for such permissions should be addressed to:
Jeremy P. Tarcher, Inc.
5858 Wilshire Blvd., Suite 200
Los Angeles, CA 90036
Published simultaneously in Canada

Library of Congress Cataloging-in-Publication Data

Janiger, Oscar.
A different kind of healing : doctors speak candidly about their
successes with alternative medicine / Oscar Janiger and Philip Goldberg.
p.   cm.
"A Jeremy P. Tarcher/Putnam Book."
Includes index.
ISBN 0-87477-728-3 (acid-free paper)
1. Alternative medicine.   2. Physicians—United States—
Interviews.   I. Goldberg, Philip, date.   II. Title.
R733J3   1993   92-37215 CIP
615.5—dc20

Printed in the United States of America
1   2   3   4   5   6   7   8   9   10

This book is printed on acid-free paper.
∞

To those dedicated physicians
who work selflessly
for the welfare of
their patients

CONTENTS

ACKNOWLEDGMENTS

We would like to thank the following people for their contributions to this book:

Jeremy Tarcher, for initiating the project and staying with it through all the changes.

Daniel Kaufman, for serving as a catalyst when the project had stalled.

Rick Benzel, for his enthusiasm and meticulous editing.

Ken Katsura and Erika Schickel, for their excellent work transcribing interviews.

Virginia D. Berg, for her diligent organizational efforts during the interview phase and her editorial assistance during the writing and rewriting phases.

Jane Brodie and Kathleen Delaney, for their steadfast personal support.

And all the doctors who gave so generously of their time and knowledge, and allowed us to use their voices.

A Different Kind of Healing

PROLOGUE

This book originated in a moment of desperation one day some years ago. One afternoon I received a phone call from a polite, cheerful woman who asked how she should introduce my speech. I panicked; I had completely forgotten my commitment to speak at a local medical society banquet that very evening. Mumbling something about wanting my topic to be a surprise, I dashed off to dress for the occasion.

As I drove to the banquet, I searched my mind for a suitable subject. If I didn't think of something quickly, my speech would be as big a surprise to me as to my audience. None of my choices seemed particularly attractive; I disliked warmed-over lecture subjects almost as much as leftover food. Then I seized upon an intriguing idea. For some reason—perhaps because I was feeling a cold coming on and wished I were home in bed—it occurred to me that in all my reading I had never seen a comprehensive review of how physicians treated *themselves* when they became ill. There had been interesting personal accounts of doctors cast in the role of patients, but these were stories of exceptional people in uncommon circumstances. I began to reflect on how ordinary physicians dealt with their own maladies.

I suspected that when doctors were ill they might explore the depths of their medical experience for unusual approaches. In extreme situations our minds tend to reach out for novel solutions and generate ideas that would not arise under ordinary conditions. Also, I reasoned, a doctor treating himself would have greater latitude for invention; he would not be restrained by the patient's resistance or an insurance carrier's refusal to cover an unconventional remedy.

Having spent over forty years in their company, I was under no illusions about the creativity of doctors. Genuine innovators are as rare in medicine as in any other field, perhaps even *more* rare, since the principal maxim of the physician's code—"Above all else, do no harm"—imposes exceptional restraints. By virtue of their training, doctors are cautious and circumspect. Nevertheless, I expected that when treating themselves or their families, they might display some inventive panache.

At the podium that evening I suggested that investigating this hypothesis might yield a wealth of priceless information. In a sense, doctors are sleuths. Over time they accumulate vast repositories of hunches, inferences, and skilled observations. Hence, I told my audience, if we were to ask practitioners about their private medical practices, we might tap into a reservoir of accumulated wisdom that would otherwise be buried with the physicians.

I laced my speech with historical anecdotes from my teaching days and told of breakthroughs that occurred when physicians used themselves as guinea pigs or fell victim to the diseases they were studying. In 1800, for example, Benjamin Waterhouse introduced the new technique of vaccination to the United States by injecting his own son—just as Edward Jenner had done in England. At great personal risk, James Y. Simpson spent night after night inhaling chemical vapors in search of an anesthetic suitable for use in childbirth. In order to determine the cause of yellow fever, James Carroll, Walter Reed, and others allowed themselves to be bitten by mosquitoes believed to be carriers of the deadly disease. This continuing legacy of courage and inventiveness, I believed, supported my hypothesis.

As it happens, present at the banquet that evening was the man who would end up publishing this book, Jeremy Tarcher. Fascinated by the issues I had raised, Jeremy invited me to lunch to discuss them further. At lunch he handed me a check. He said the money was to help cover expenses for a pilot research project about how doctors treat themselves. I politely declined. After more than forty years in private practice, hospitals, and universities, I had had my fill of deadlines. Jeremy's response was, "If you change your mind, cash the check."

Faced with such unexpected support, I could not resist. I cashed the check.

Having decided to take up the challenge, I decided to try for some degree of objectivity and to collect a representative sample of physicians. I divided Los Angeles into geographical areas and selected physicians at random from the phone directory. The resulting sample of two hundred doctors included men and women whose professional experience ranged from a few years to four decades, and whose practices ran the gamut from small neighborhood offices to leading universities and hospitals. Most were family practitioners, but a generous number of internists, gynecologists, cardiologists, and other specialists were included. I trained a trio of bright, well-educated research assistants to conduct the interviews, which were later transcribed and coded.

At first glance, the results were, to put it mildly, disappointing. It turned out that the doctors we interviewed (and, we can reasonably extrapolate, doctors in general) did not, when ill, call upon a private treasure trove of remedies. They treated themselves just as they would an ordinary patient with the same condition. That is, if they treated themselves at all. Many respondents said they adhered to the oft-repeated adage that anyone who treats himself has a fool for a patient. Nor were they inclined to treat close family members, except in emergencies or for common complaints such as a headache or cold. They felt they could not be sufficiently objective with a spouse, parent, or child. Only in a few instances did we get an anecdote reflecting what we were looking for: an unconventional treatment that the doctors used only on themselves, not their patients. That handful of exceptions, which appear in this book, represented only a dim glimmer of confirmation for my speculation the night of the banquet.

My initial disappointment was short-lived, however, for the survey serendipitously yielded treasures of a more valuable kind. Fortunately, I had allowed for a certain latitude in the interviews that permitted the doctors to expound on another topic of abiding interest: how their ideas and private practices had changed over the course of their careers. While most responses were anticipated, a number of those queried were eager to discuss issues like the state of contemporary medicine, the shortcomings of medical training, and the various forces compelling and restraining change. Sprinkled into the dialogues were fascinating anecdotes about unusual experiences with patients and pivotal moments in their own careers. Most of these stories were about their use of unconventional treatments—not on themselves, as we had hoped for, but on their patients.

The subject of nontraditional healing practices had also been of particular interest to me over the years. Early in my career, I sought out patients who had recovered from serious illnesses in order to hear what they thought had made them get better. Their accounts included such nonmedical elements as prayer, will power, meditation, and the support of loved ones. I also spent time with native healers in various cultures and had come to respect their skills. In the early seventies, convinced that the medical community might learn a great deal by widening its range of inquiry, I accepted an appointment as Chairman of the Research Committee of the Holmes Center for Research in Holistic Healing, a nonprofit foundation that provided grants for the scientific investigation of nonconventional medical practices. For over a decade, we awarded tens of thousands of dollars and served as an information clearing house for health professionals and interested laypersons. Several of those grantees went on to make significant contributions to the practice of medicine.

It was, therefore, with growing interest that I read the results of our initial round of interviews. The responses confirmed two of my personal observations. First, doctors are considerably more diverse in temperament and personality than is commonly appreciated. We want our healers to be uniformly skilled and efficient, with personalities cloned from Dr. Kildare and Marcus Welby. But doctors come in many modes: compassionate and cold; well-rounded and narrow-visioned; conservatives who cling to established values and mavericks who challenge conventional wisdom; creative visionaries and assembly-line robots. These personal differences, which were reflected in our interviews, certainly affect the course and outcome of individual patient's treatment.

The interviews also confirmed my belief that medical practice is in the throes of a major transformation. This has been noted by many observers, but it was instructive to see it spelled out in the words of ordinary physicians describing their routine activities, unusual approaches, and private thoughts. While our sample is statistically small, my overall impression is that the doctors expressed a representative range of opinions. At one extreme were those to whom deviation from the mainstream was unthinkable and who expressed an almost smug satisfaction with the status quo. At the other pole were those whose philosophies and practices had undergone radical departures from the norm, to the extent of advocating revolutionary change. In between were the majority of our respondents, who provided the biggest surprise.

I found that many of the attitudes and practices that were regarded as radical in my days at the Holmes Center had since filtered into the mainstream. I refer to certain premises of the holistic health movement: that mental and spiritual factors can influence the disease process, that drugs and surgery are frequently overused, that the human touch is vital in the doctor-patient relationship, and that alternative healing methods can be of significant value. Our interviews suggested that mainstream doctors are not as adverse to unconventional practices as they were ten years ago. At the same time, those who embrace the unorthodox appear to be more conciliatory toward the establishment. The radicals, it seems, have softened their stance as they accumulated experience and credibility, while conservatives yielded ground in the face of further understanding and empirical evidence.

This is precisely the picture one would expect for an institution in the midst of change: a small number on the extreme end of either position and the majority in the center where values overlap, leaning one way or the other.

Inspired by the broad picture painted by the interviews and the illuminating candor of the stories and anecdotes, I decided that a book would indeed be a worthwhile endeavor. I joined forces with my coauthor, who had written extensively about health issues, and together we decided to revitalize the original material. We returned to some of the original two hundred respondents for additional information. In addition, we embarked upon a fresh round of interviews with doctors who had been referred to us by colleagues, thereby extending our reach to other parts of the country. In all, two hundred and fifty doctors were queried.

As finally constituted, I believe that the book presents a doctor's eye view—an oral history, if you will—of an important transitional period in the history of Western medicine, from a prescribed and somewhat inflexible system to one that is more exploratory and open to different concepts and procedures.

The results in this book are more impressionistic than scientific, and we present the information here mainly through the anecdotes and case histories of our interviewees. We have extracted from a huge pile of transcripts the most interesting accounts and provocative ideas, including some that lie in a gray area of medicine—neither patently right nor wrong, but largely unproven. Nonetheless, it is important to note that the material quoted was voiced by physicians with rigorous academic training and a good deal of clinical experience. These M.D.s could have safely selected any conventional therapy or treatment available for a patient, yet they occasionally felt that an alternative treatment was more appropriate or offered a greater chance of success. Admittedly, unconventional ideas comprise a far greater portion of the book than they did the actual interviews, yet I am convinced their overall tenor is consistent with the changing views of a sizeable number of physicians.

Here, then, are the most unusual experiences in mainstream medicine, along with the radical, sometimes bizarre, ideas of those on the periphery of the profession. No names are included. Since many physicians made anonymity a condition of their participation, we decided to name no one rather than only those who would permit it.

The first chapter provides a historical perspective, combining my own views with comments from our doctors. The last two chapters are handled in much the same manner, only looking toward the future rather than the past; the doctors we interviewed had much to say about where they thought medicine should go and how future doctors ought to be trained. The chapters in between focus mainly on our doctors' firsthand experiences with methods of healing they did not learn about in the course of their training but acquired in various ways subsequently.

One of my purposes in presenting the material in this manner is to give physicians an opportunity to share with colleagues their clinical experiences involving unusual remedies and unorthodox therapies. Doctors are deluged as never before with information—in journals, newsletters, computer files, advertising, even a special radio band and cable television station—but the opportunity to exchange valuable shop talk with peers has declined. They tend to work long hours, often under such intense conditions that opportunities for the exchange of ideas are limited. The kind of informal observations presented here seldom get written up in professional journals, and most doctors have neither the inclination nor the resources to subject their ideas to formal experimentation. I hope that the book will encourage further dialogue and more research into unconventional practices.

My second reason is clearly to inform the public as to the variety and scope of treatment possibilities and the slowly evolving acceptability of alternative medicine. I am committed to the notion that medicine has many divergent aspects, that it is a veritable mansion with many rooms. I believe that healing often follows what I call the "idiosyncratic rule," which refers to the unique relationship an individual has with his illness, meaning that each of us reacts and responds to an illness and its treatment in his own, and sometimes unpredictable, ways. I have tried to lend insight into how doctors think and to describe alternative treatments being used by some well-trained physicians. As a result, I hope you, the reader, will be better prepared to choose among the variety of medical services available and become a better health-care consumer.

However, I must also emphasize that the inclusion of information in this book in no way constitutes an endorsement for applying that treatment to any individual. The treatments you will read about were entirely dependent upon the individual patient and doctor involved. In fact, no doctor we interviewed would discuss the specific dosages of the medicines, supplements or remedies he used, since it is obviously foolhardy to extrapolate one patient's treatment to another without knowing the specifics of each individual's situation. Especially if you are experiencing a serious health crisis, I urge you to consult your personal physician about any of the remedies or treatments mentioned that you feel might be of benefit to you.

It is my hope that you will come away from this book with a glimpse into the ferment of diverse ideas that is changing the face of medicine, plus a better understanding of the professionals to whom you entrust your health.

CHAPTER 1

THE EVOLUTION OF MODERN MEDICINE

In 1910, the Carnegie Foundation for the Advancement of Teaching published a report entitled *Medical Education in the United States and Canada*. The survey, which came to be known as the Flexner Report after its author, Abraham Flexner, was a defining event in the history of American medicine.

At the time, a kind of anarchy reigned. A wide variety of philosophies and practices competed for favor, with cadres of practitioners advocating each. Schools offered training that reflected vastly different approaches, from science-based curricula at prestigious universities to apprenticeship programs with a handful of disciples. All turned out graduates who could obtain licenses and call themselves doctors. Naturally, graduates of reputable institutions such as Harvard and Johns Hopkins had an advantage in the marketplace over people from the No-Name School of Applied Therapy, but politically and legally there was little distinction.

Concluding that the system was in sad disarray and most schools shamefully deficient, the Flexner Report recommended a system of standardized training, licensing, and regulation. Subsequently, schools that met the Flexner standards were accredited and the others were disqualified. In the ensuing years, nearly half the medical schools in North America were closed and a reported $600,000,000 was spent to make medical education science-based and research-oriented. It was a milestone in the attempt to elevate healing from a somewhat unpredictable art to a scientifically oriented practice.

The impact was enormous, and it reverberated beyond its original intentions. Now only graduates of the newly accredited schools were granted the degree of Medical Doctor and allowed to apply for membership in the American Medical Association, which became the principal standard-bearer of the Flexner principles. As a result of this winnowing process, the philosophies and practices associated with approved institutions were legitimized. Acceptable medicine became that which conformed to the standards of science, while ideas and practices associated with unaccredited schools were denigrated and strict limits imposed on their practitioners.

It could scarcely have been appreciated at the time, but in throwing out the proverbial dirty bathwater of quacks and charlatans, the healing arts also lost a few babies that might have been worth salvaging. Instead of objectively seeking out what might be valuable in osteopathy, chiropractic, naturopathy, homeopathy, and the like, authorities lumped them together with the dangerous and dispensable. Thus, alternatives that might have contributed something worthwhile were stigmatized and relegated to the sidelines of medicine. Further, the criteria for what constitutes acceptable medicine and who shall be granted the status of legitimate physician began to be defined along political and jurisdictional lines. The issue became who is entitled to do what as opposed to who and what is good at helping sick people get better.

The supremacy of rational-empirical medicine—which has also come to be called allopathic or Western medicine—was justified by history. More than a hundred years earlier, the practice of vaccination and the early science of immunology ushered in a new era in health care. That same period witnessed two other major advances: sanitation reform, with its sewage systems, clean water supplies, sterilization procedures, widespread use of soap and other weapons against the filth that spread disease; and the observations of Rudolf Virchow, Louis Pasteur, and others that led to the concept of cellular pathology and the germ theory of disease. This theory held that illness was caused when a specific agent—a bacterium or other microorganism— invaded the body. It was further assumed that a cure could be effected by destroying or neutralizing the infecting agent. This was further verified by the work of German bacteriologist Robert Koch, who was able to isolate and grow the anthrax bacillus in pure culture and reproduce the disease in animals. The new approach was perfectly suited to the treatment of virulent afflictions that had been ravaging Europe and America—infectious diseases such as bubonic plague, cholera, typhoid fever, diphtheria, and smallpox.

Strengthened by the new reforms and the introduction of new instruments, medical science rolled like a juggernaut through the first half of the century, crushing one microbe after another until, in the Western world at least, a large number of infectious diseases that had tormented our ancestors were virtually conquered. With each success came greater status, power, and authority. Science-based medicine became the sine qua non; funding for hospitals, clinics, and research were channeled almost exclusively toward institutions that embodied the new mainstream, and the M.D. degree became a symbol of respectability and competence. By World War II, the title of "doctor" had reached the apogee of trustworthiness and honor. To wary observers, however, it had also come to stand for arrogance and elitism. Excluding everything that did not fit under the strict rubric of scientific medicine, the establishment, as represented by the American Medical Association, was accused of being overly concerned with protecting the privileges of insiders at the expense of public health.

On the theoretical level, a trend had been established that attempted to fit all diseases into the procrustean bed of scientific allopathy. In a Greek legend, Procrustes was a robber who placed people on an iron bed. If the person were too long, Procrustes chopped off his overhanging parts; if he were too short, the guest was stretched until he filled the bed. Analogously, the assumption that every disease would fit comfortably into the conceptual framework that accommodated infectious disease proved to be a fallacy. As time went on, physicians were forced to acknowledge that many diseases did not suit their model of causality. These included the various forms of arthritis and arteriosclerosis as well as cancer, hypertension, and immuno-suppressive diseases, which appeared to have multiple causes. These illnesses became more prevalent as the average life span was increased.

Change was further hastened by the gradual validation of an ancient notion that mental and emotional conditions can affect the course of disease. This assertion had been voiced as far back as biblical times, but it was given little official notice until the delineation of psychosomatic illness after the First World War. Mainstream physicians had tended to dismiss psychological factors as irrelevant or insignificant in the course of an individual's physical illness, and if they acknowledged them at all, it was to "blame" the patient's attitude or lifestyle as causal. They condescendingly used terms like "placebo," "spontaneous remission," and the "power of suggestion," even when the psychological impact was positive, to shrug off phenomena they could not explain. But, as evidence accumulated, it became more and more difficult to ignore the obvious: the mind contributes to both the cause and cure of disease. Gradually, psychiatrists, who had been limited to the treatment of mental illness, were brought into the fold by bolder colleagues in other specialties who began to consult them about patients who exhibited "unusual" or "unexplainable" symptoms.

Also, about this time, Hans Selye and others were documenting their observations that the clinical effect of stress was mediated by our behavior, attitudes, and emotions. It was becoming evident that excessive stress could weaken the body and its defenses against illness. Here was accumulating evidence that we were not just fighting viruses and bacteria but the organism's inherent liability to stress compounded by the increasing toxicity of the environment. Also, the notion of resistance was being redefined by studies of the role of heredity on disease, the specialized functions of the immune system, and our growing understanding of the complex nature of the response to disease and treatment. Clearly, susceptibility to disease entailed the patient's genetic makeup plus a wide range of environmental factors that were previously considered peripheral to the concerns of medical science.

THE WOODSTOCK GENERATION

By the 1960s, the theoretical model on which modern medicine had been erected was being seriously challenged, and the impulse to question prevailing wisdom was compounded by social forces. In keeping with the spirit of the times, segments of the population realized that medicine was as imperfect as other institutions. Along with authority figures from schoolteachers to presidents, doctors found their pedestals shaking beneath their feet. Medicine was faulted for becoming depersonalized, a charge stemming from spiraling costs, reliance on technology at the expense of the human touch, bureaucracies made necessary by hospital-based treatment and third-party reimbursement, the sudden preponderance of specialists, and the near extinction of the wise, caring family doctor who knew his patients intimately and attended them from cradle to grave.

Even highly successful treatment modalities came under fire. Critics charged that surgery was performed too often where less costly, less risky alternatives might be as effective. Miracle drugs turned out to have side effects that were sometimes as bad as the illnesses they were designed to combat. Doctors were faulted for being disease-centered rather than person- and health-centered. For many disorders, treatments provided only temporary relief by suppressing symptoms; they could not eliminate the underlying causes or prevent the outbreak of disease.

None of this was lost on physicians. In fact, it was frequently doctors themselves who led the charge and proffered the most compelling arguments. Many physicians grew increasingly disaffected and found less gratification in their practices, a trend that culminated in a recent poll that indicated that forty percent of American doctors would choose other professions if they had it to do all over again. Furthermore, the sixties' ethos of experimentation and individuality led many doctors, the young in particular, to search for alternatives outside the narrow limits of accepted practice. Some made radical changes in their professional orientations. The following are illustrative tales drawn from the interviews we did for this book:

"I was traveling around before beginning medical school, and I found myself in Paris in 1968, at the time of the student riots. After one of the big demonstrations, about four in the morning, someone thrust under my nose a book about acupuncture. It had some very curious photographs. On the cover was a face with needles sticking out of it. It seemed to me bizarre, exotic, and somehow terribly fascinating. I bought the book, read it, and put it away as something to follow up on sometime."

His follow-up came five years later, when he was unable to decide on a specialty. "I was waiting for a specialty to identify itself with a display of fireworks or some cosmic announcement that this was my path. I was well trained, I performed my duties in emergency rooms and clinics, but there was no click with a specialty. So I went to France to study, and I looked into acupuncture, which was not considered new or strange in Europe." Pursuing his interest on breaks from his residency, he eventually featured acupuncture when he went into private practice. "I'm a family practitioner. I orient my work responsibly around the basic principles of good medicine. I see a broad clientele, from pediatrics to geriatrics, but the main reason people come to see me is acupuncture."

Another physician who was influenced by the spirit of the sixties started as a student with an interest in Zen Buddhism. "I was open to anything different, and I just kept adding on over time. When I was in medical school, my roommates and I became macrobiotic. After my internship, I got involved with a spiritual group and moved to Hawaii, where I worked in a hospital by day and spent my evenings studying esoteric things."

A few years later, he heard that the roommate who got him into macrobiotics was now a physician. "He was doing weird stuff connected to external factors that influence people's health. He got me interested in the environmental aspect—different kinds of allergies, chemical and electrical exposure, stress, family dynamics. So I took a course and started working in that area a year or two after I opened my office." He stated that the spiritual studies he began in the sixties still provide him with a larger perspective: "The whole sense of movement and flow and energy—that aspect of Eastern thought inspired me, and I was moved by the idea of expanded consciousness and a greater connection to the world. I think one reason my patients get better is the way I relate to them—dealing with their problems consciously, and trying to get them to go beyond defending their egos and to reflect upon a greater sense of self."

For another child of the sixties her formative experience preceded her decision to enter medicine: "I was a student traveling through Europe. I had dropped out of college and had no idea what I wanted to do with my life. I worked on a biodynamic farm for a while. It was part of Rudolph Steiner's work, a metaphysical system of agriculture meant to bring higher energies into the plants and support the growth of consciousness. I became totally enamored of herbalism. Then I became an exchange student at a homeopathic hospital in Germany. I wasn't even thinking of being a doctor, it was all just curiosity. I worked in the kitchen for a while. They were vegetarians using a lot of whole grains. Then I worked as a nurse's aid. Patients got all sorts of treatments—homeopathy, baths, rubdowns with oil, art and music therapy, movement therapy, a multidimensional program.

"I can't tell you that I saw miraculous cures, but I was introduced to the fact that there are many different ways medicine can be practiced. I realized that if I had a choice in how I or a close family member would be treated, I wouldn't want it to be the way I'd seen it done in America, especially because the metaphysical approach was very real to me." She returned to the U.S. and eventually entered medical school, where she often felt like an outsider. But she persevered and now supplements conventional procedures with alternative modalities.

Young physicians such as the ones just quoted went on to become the vanguard of an influential new movement. In the early 1970s, a group of doctors launched what came to be called "the holistic health movement." The rebels exhorted colleagues to focus not on disease as such, but on the "whole person," not just on the body but on mind, spirit, and environment as they impact on health. They called for disease prevention and the promotion of maximum "wellness." They advocated more "natural" modes of treatment, and searched for them outside the usual medical repertoire—in foreign cultures, folk remedies, and esoteric sources. They also urged patients to assume a more active role in the prevention and treatment of disease through changes in their attitude and lifestyle.

As might be expected, the radicals were denounced by the mainstream as quacks and turncoats. Rather than approach these new ideas in the spirit of open inquiry, many opponents chose to close ranks and defend their turf, concluding a priori that the mavericks were not worthy of consideration. Some in the avant-garde were prosecuted by courts or censured by medical societies. More thoughtful critics argued that some of the new-wave doctors were as dogmatic and elitist as the establishment they deplored, embracing unproven treatments that fit their ideology while rejecting proven scientific advances. Others faulted them for betraying their holistic credo by specializing in one faddish practice or another. Most members of the holistic movement, however, were responsible physicians searching ardently for effective alternatives. Over time, through a kind of selective infiltration, the useful information they unearthed managed to cross the barriers of antagonism and stimulate needed changes in medical thought.

The holistic movement has also made inroads among medical consumers. A 1991 poll by *Time* magazine found that thirty percent of those questioned had tried some form of alternative therapy. The same poll found that eighty-four percent of that group would return to unconventional practitioners. Of those who had *not* sought alternative treatments, fully sixty-two percent said they would do so if conventional medicine were to fail them.

A number of the physicians we interviewed had been early converts to the holistic movement. Some radically altered their careers; most modified their practices to a limited degree, selectively integrating new ideas into an otherwise conventional practice. We will hear from many of these doctors throughout the book.

HOW INERTIA GIVES WAY TO CHANGE

New ideas find their way to doctors through a variety of means. Mainstream drugs and technologies are brought to their attention through professional journals, magazines, conferences, and the voluminous mail sent out by manufacturers. Less conventional ideas filter in by way of the occasional article, professional and social contacts with colleagues, serendipitous personal experiences, or the urging of singular patients. Our interviews yielded examples of all of these. But more interesting than their contact with new ideas is why some doctors are actually influenced by them.

Some people are willing to entertain concepts that others disregard out of hand as unworthy or threatening. Some minds are flexible, curious, tolerant of ambiguity, and willing to question their own assumptions, while others resist new ideas like the body does a virus. Nothing illustrates these differences as well as doctors' reactions to cases of remarkable healing. Patients frequently defy our expectations: diseases improve sooner than our diagnoses predict, symptoms regarded as intractable suddenly disappear, people live on despite conditions that are considered terminal, cures are effected by methods that don't fit our theories. Faced with such phenomena, one kind of physician will shrug them off, attributing them to spontaneous remission, placebo, coincidence, or the power of suggestion, as if these labels should settle all further inquiries.

Other doctors faced with inexplicable events find their curiosity aroused, particularly when the events occur more than once. To them, an anomaly repeatedly observed is not an aberration but a pattern; spontaneous remissions are unexplained phenomena that demand fresh theories; a placebo is not a medical parlor trick but evidence that faith and trust can have potent physiological consequences; unorthodox remedies are not necessarily fraudulent but potential additions to the medical arsenal. In short, what inspires contempt or indifference from one doctor might inspire research or bold speculation in another.

Such personality factors create a dynamic tension between proponents of change and defenders of the status quo. The push and pull of those forces is what enables any science, including medicine, to evolve. Over the course of time, however, it is pragmatism that rules. Like any profession with responsibility for the well-being of others, medicine is conservative by nature. However, the principal concern of doctors is to cure disease. Like all problem-solvers, from plumbers to presidents, if their methods come up short, they are drawn to anything that might work. Eventually, if something is shown to be efficacious, either by the weight of scientific evidence or convincing personal accounts, it will find support, first from the eager mavericks, then the pragmatists, and eventually even the grudging hard-liners.

The following statements attribute personal transformations to a variety of circumstances and influences. In the first story, a disillusioned dropout finds her way to a satisfying practice:

"At the end of two years as a medical resident, I looked around and thought, we're killing more people than we're curing, and we're not curing enough. So I said to heck with it and left. I quit my residency and sold real estate for a couple of years. But I would find myself in the office reading medical journals and thinking, have I missed something? Is my heart still in it?"

She returned to medicine under the auspices of an influential mentor: "Working for him was a real turning point. He was doing nutritional holistic medicine. He taught me a lot and sent me to conferences where I discovered a whole new world of organizations, caucuses, newsletters, and journals. It was just great. I vowed that for every single problem I would find a treatment that was not a drug. I had a whole bookcase full of 'advisors,' as I called them, and I would unashamedly, in front of a patient, say, 'Let's see what so-and-so has to say about your problem.' I would read to them and say, 'Here's the recommended dosage of Vitamin E for breast cysts. Why don't you try this?' I attracted a clientele that was interested in an M.D. who understood traditional medicine and was also willing to try something different. They didn't want to take drugs, which amazed me: they told us in medical school, don't ever offer anything besides drugs because you'll lose your patients.

"I never returned to my residency. My heart wasn't in it. When I saw how well the alternatives worked—techniques I never learned about in medical school—I couldn't go back to pushing pills and fancy drugs on people. It would be like sitting out in the sunshine and then having to go back into your cave again."

The next story was related by a Texas cardiologist whose transformation was precipitated by a mid-life crisis: "I was working from early morning till late at night, sometimes sixteen hours a day. Then one day I stopped and asked myself, 'Is this what you want to do for the rest of your life?' The answer was immediately, 'No-o-o-o!' It was almost a scream, a cry for help."

He left his practice and worked in an educational capacity. There, he received inquiries about Nathan Pritikin, who became famous in the mid-seventies by claiming that heart disease could be prevented, or even cured, with diet and exercise. "I categorically denied that any of that business was possible. It just couldn't be. Later on, I left my marriage, put all my belongings in a camper, and headed for California. I looked up Pritikin, who told me about his work. I thought, 'If he can do these things with diet, I want to know about it. If he's a charlatan, I'll soon figure it out.' So, when he offered me a job at his clinic, I accepted.

"It didn't take me long to see that he was right. I had worked in a diabetes clinic for two years, and I never saw anyone's diabetes get better. Pritikin was treating people who were on insulin and oral medication, and in a matter of days or weeks got many of them off all medicine, through a strict regimen of diet and exercise." The cardiologist went on to establish his own practice in nutritional medicine.

Another convert who started out a skeptic was an allergist whose assumptions were challenged by unconventional colleagues: "The turning point came at a conference. I was very cocky, sure that I was doing the best possible work in the world, and I listened skeptically to some fellows who were using a new method of testing and treatment called provocation neutralization. They claimed that certain substances could be allergens that were not recognized by traditional allergists. They said that legs could ache because of a milk allergy, and that headaches and depression could be caused by eating particular foods. Allergies to foods could also result in hyperactivity, aggression, and learning problems. They reported very few patients on cortisone and didn't write many prescriptions. I thought, they're lying through their teeth. I paid a visit to one of the speakers, intending to expose a fraud. I watched very carefully, and when I came home I told my husband, that man is so clever he duped me for four days."

Eventually, she tried the new approach on patients, and the results were dramatic enough to dent her skepticism: "I was very resistant to changing my practice. It took two years of going to meetings and checking and investigating before I finally said to myself, 'This method is better. You've got to change your practice, in spite of what everybody says.' It's far more time-consuming, but much more effective. I could never go back to practicing the old way."

For some physicians, the experience of being a patient was pivotal. The following excerpt describes how a personal illness led to the decision to go into medicine: "I had been a very sick kid for years. I was raised on erythromycin as if it were a vitamin. I had ear infections, allergies, sinus infections, sore throats. I was depressed, fatigued, thin, and pale. I had my tonsils out and my adenoids removed, and I'd grown up on antibiotics, so my bowels were a wreck. One morning I woke up sick and angry and I looked in the mirror and said, 'I am sick of being sick!' I was seventeen or eighteen and I set out to discover what it would take for me to be healthy."

Embarking on a typical 1970s journey of self-exploration, he became a vegetarian, meditated, practiced yoga, and explored Gestalt therapy and transactional analysis. Of his experimentation, he said: "It helped me to get away from what I was taught and to see other possibilities." Later, having improved his own condition, he decided to share what he had learned by going to medical school and supplementing his training by studying then-offbeat practices such as biofeedback, acupuncture, and hypnotherapy. "If you had asked me a year before if I wanted to be a doctor, I'd have said, 'No way!' I'd grown up disliking doctors."

A surprising number of respondents said they were introduced to new treatments by patients. The attitude of such doctors, as opposed to those who blithely dismissed unorthodox ideas as naive, is captured in this statement by a veteran internist: "If there's one thing I've learned in my twenty-one years in medicine, it's that I can't cure all diseases. There are some conditions I just can't help, and if the patient comes up with something he thinks is helping him, and it's not harmful, good God, let him use it, whether it really works or not. An arthritis patient of mine was drinking some weird mixture of gelatin and blueberries. I wondered if there might be some chemical compound in that mixture that really had some effect on the cartilage and joints that we don't know about yet. Maybe these people aren't really crazy, and if they say it makes them feel better, why do I have any right to tell them it's hogwash as long as it doesn't stand in the way of a treatment that I know to be effective?"

The next two stories are from doctors who were influenced by unusual patients. First, a psychiatrist recalls a challenge from a young patient: "She was eighteen. Her father insisted that she see me because she was doing a lot of drugs. At one point, she was getting a lot better, but she said, 'I'm able to get off drugs because I'm meditating. That's what's healing me. You think it's your therapy, but it isn't. It's my meditation."

"I asked her to tell me more, and she said, 'I can't tell you what it's about. I dare you to go over and see for yourself.' She was a very wise eighteen-year-old. I was skeptical, but I was also curious, so I tried it. I had a very positive experience the first time I meditated. It was remarkable. My whole life changed. First, I noticed that I was healing myself. I used to regularly sprain my ankle playing tennis. Almost every month I would be laid up for a week with a swollen ankle. The next time it happened, I went upstairs to meditate, and when I came down, I realized that I was bounding down the stairs, the swelling in the ankle had gone down and it wasn't sore. I was totally amazed." The experience led her to study a variety of meditation and visualization techniques, which she still uses with patients afflicted with everything from sexual problems to cancer.

In the next story, an insistent patient launches a family physician into a controversial career change: "I started out doing the full gamut of family practice. One of my patients was a housewife who had been under treatment for depression. I referred her to a psychoanalyst and gave her drugs—Miltown and amphetamines to elevate her mood.

"Well, after ten years of this, she came in one day with a woman's magazine and said, 'I just read this article. You've been treating me for the wrong problem. I'm not depressed. I have low blood sugar.' I said, 'Come on!' But she made me read the article. It said that hypoglycemia was very common and doctors didn't often recognize that it causes fatigue, depression, anxiety, and headaches—the most outrageous bunch of nonsense. I told the patient it was ridiculous, but she said, 'I know that's my problem. Can't I take a glucose tolerance test?'

"I couldn't think of any reason to say no, so she went to the local hospital and took a six-hour glucose tolerance test. Well, she scared the technician half to death. She had palpitations and almost passed out. When I looked at the results, I told her that she certainly did have low blood sugar, but I was at a loss as to how to treat it. She said that the article mentioned a place to contact for professional literature. I got the literature and read it, but I was very defensive and told the patient, 'This is too much to swallow. I'm not going to get involved.' But she begged me to visit one of the doctors mentioned in the article.

"Out of respect for this long-standing patient, I spent a day with one of those doctors. I spoke to patients who swore they had been basket cases and their lives had been turned around without antidepressants or tranquilizers—just a change of diet, some exercise, vitamins, and injections of adrenal cortical extract. I was really stunned. I came back with a printed diet and a list of vitamins, and I gave them to my patient to see what would happen. She did magnificently. She felt better than she ever felt. My reaction was, she really believes in this; it's just an expensive placebo."

He remained skeptical until he connected her medical problem with one in his own family: "My daughter was fourteen at the time and had changed from the child I had known. She was chronically tired. She was coming home from school and taking naps. She had headaches all the time. She was bitchy and irritable and couldn't concentrate on her homework. We took her to a psychiatrist, who said it was a typical adolescent rebellion syndrome. He wanted to see her a couple of times a week. Then I remembered the low blood sugar. I thought, let's do a glucose tolerance test. It was normal according to everything I'd learned in medical school, but not according to the standards of the Hypoglycemia Foundation. I put her on a hypoglyce-

mic diet of high protein with frequent feeding and no refined carbohy-
drates.

"In about three weeks the change in her energy and joie de vivre
was incredible. She stopped having headaches, was studying again, and
all her physical symptoms were resolved. It really got to me because
I was responsible for her misery. I was her father, a doctor, and I raised
her on this terrible diet. I should have known better. I felt it was a
condemnation of the medical training I had followed all those years."
He went on to specialize in nutritional medicine and other alternative
practices, earning the enmity of his local medical board.

In a number of instances, change was precipitated by extraordinary
personal experiences. The next two excerpts recall incidents of such
intense anguish that the doctors felt compelled to rethink their approach to their profession. Each took place in inner city emergency
rooms:

"It was about three or four in the morning. I was exhausted and
irritable. They wheeled in this guy who looked like he'd had a stroke.
His blood pressure was way up and he was incoherent. I had to look
through the pupil of his eye to see if I could get some clues about what
was going on. But he kept moving around. I started to get rough with
him, trying to hold him still, but he kept moving, and I got rougher
and rougher, and finally he looked up at me and said, 'Why are you
torturing me?'

"I said, 'I'm trying to help you, goddamn it! Keep your head still.'
Well, that Sunday while I was driving, I heard those words: 'Why are
you torturing me?' I felt they were telling me there's something
terribly wrong. What's happening to me?"

He concluded that the humanitarian values that had led him to
pursue a medical career had been beaten out of him by the grind of
training and practice: "I decided to take some time off, to get some rest
and do some serious thinking. That's when I chose to check out
holistic medicine." He went on to develop a family practice that
features an eclectic mix of treatments and close ties to his patients.

In the next story, a small-town doctor with a conventional practice remembers a pivotal moment during an emergency room rotation: "I arrived for my shift one morning at seven o'clock, and the doctor who was signing out said, 'There's a guy over there in pajamas who had a mild sleeping pill overdose. He's ready to go home. Check him out.'

"I talked to the man. He told me he'd had trouble sleeping and had taken some pills. He came to the emergency room because he was feeling a little unsteady, a bit off the wall. I said, 'You weren't trying to kill yourself, were you?' He said, 'Oh, no, I was just having trouble sleeping.' So I discharged him. I had a lot of patients to see, so I kind of shined him off in the heat of the moment and promptly forgot about him.

"About two o'clock that afternoon, the doors flew open and the medics came racing down the hall with a body on a gurney, and I noticed out of the corner of my eye that the patient's pajamas were the same ones I'd seen on the guy I sent home a few hours before. He had a gunshot wound in his abdomen. He was bleeding heavily, and they were trying to get him stabilized. I sidled up to him and said, 'You told me you weren't trying to kill yourself.' He said, 'I guess I was lying.'

"He died. He had shot himself in the abdomen. I remember feeling so strange. How did I miss it? There were things that suggested he wasn't just taking an occasional sleeping pill at night. He was depressed. He was about sixty years old and still living with his mother. Should I have had him see the psychiatrist? Would that have made a difference? Eighteen years later I can remember the scene with crystal clarity. I think the patient picked up the implication that I didn't want to be bothered, that I was busy and he was in my way, so his natural reaction was, 'Oh, no, I wasn't trying to kill myself.' He wasn't getting the support he needed to reveal the truth."

The experience made the doctor question his training: "I was taught that an effective clinician can't be emotionally involved, that you have to stand off from the patient and be the white-coat university picture of the doctor. The process is not designed to support feelings. It makes you an effective clinician in a narrow way—very physiological, very biological. Medical school takes people, some of whom have a decent liberal arts education, and turns them into quasi-scientists."

Haunted by the memory of that suicide, he said, he works hard to offer his patients empathy: "I try to be as open-ended as possible when I talk to them. I've learned to tune in to what the patient is *not* telling me. The more I pay attention to all aspects of the patient's life, the more I understand the person, the better I can tailor my approach to him." As we shall see in later chapters, his comments were mirrored by a remarkable number of physicians who, despite otherwise divergent views, despaired that modern medicine has lost the human touch that had traditionally been attributed to the village doctor or medicine man.

A SNAPSHOT OF WHERE WE ARE

As is usually the case when prevailing ideas clash and an institution muddles through a period of transition, establishment doctors and their less conventional colleagues still exist in a state of dynamic tension. But the boundaries have dissolved considerably, and the critics have managed to stimulate much-needed change. For example, complaints that medicine does not pay enough attention to preventive measures accelerated the trend in which the risk factors associated with various disorders are identified and advanced diagnostic tools ascertain the early warning signs of disease. The same critics also hastened efforts to educate the public about mental and physical stress, smoking, drinking, and other destructive lifestyle factors. Research on diet, the immune system, the brain's role in mediating health, and the impact of noxious elements in the environment was given added impetus by the ideological conflict between the nontraditional camp and the mainstream.

With respect to actual practice, many treatment approaches that were, not long ago, regarded as radical have inched their way into established practice. It is no longer considered odd, for example, to teach a patient ways to reduce stress, or issue nutritional advice that goes beyond official recommendations, or to evaluate a patient's psychological condition when treating a physical disorder. Our interviews clearly suggest that the classic model of change, in which the clash of thesis and antithesis invariably leads to a new synthesis, is being followed by contemporary medicine.

At the same time, the interviews indicate that most unorthodox physicians are not as contemptuous of conventional medicine as they once seemed to be. Virtually all the unorthodox practitioners we spoke to took pains to emphasize that they do not entirely eschew drugs, surgery, and other traditional procedures, even if they prescribe them less frequently than their colleagues or regard them as treatments of last resort. Here are some typically conciliatory statements from doctors whose orientation places them squarely in the alternative group:

"By conventional standards, I may seem unconventional, but by unconventional standards, I'm very conventional. I try to form a bridge between the poles of alternative medicine and orthodox practice. Some of my patients may go to great lengths to deny the value of a procedure because of some fixed ideas. I'm reminded of one with severe back pain who went from one healer to another in search of a natural cure, only to have her pain get worse. I told her to see an orthopedic surgeon, and he found a serious disk impairment. She had surgery, and is presently free of pain."

Said a cardiologist who specializes in diet, exercise, and psychotherapy: "There are two extremes: doing a bypass when it's not needed, and *not* doing a bypass when it *is* needed. I've seen patients who are so anti-medicine that although they come in with severe chest pain and can't walk across the room, they still won't take anything. I try to be eclectic. I prescribe blood pressure medication where appropriate, especially for people with intermittent stress, like an accountant at tax time. The difference is, I don't see it as a first-line treatment."

Here is a doctor who practices homeopathy but has not entirely forsaken his traditional education: "I use my allopathic training every day. For instance, a woman called me to make an appointment. She said she was bleeding from the nipple. I said, 'Before I see you, you need to see Dr. So-and-So and let him examine your breast and do a mammogram. Bleeding from the nipple is cancer until proven otherwise.' I had another lady who came with an unusual kind of diarrhea. I gave her a few remedies that should have cured it, but they didn't, so I sent her to a gastroenterologist to rule out cancer of the colon."

One alternative doctor said his arrogance was knocked out of him by a dramatic incident in a holistic clinic: "A big, rough-looking guy came in with back pain. I manipulated him with a chiropractic technique, and he felt somewhat better. When I didn't hear back from him, I called and asked how he'd been. I was feeling pompous. I was ready to hear that he was doing great. He said, 'You jerk! I had a kidney stone.' I had missed it totally. It would have been a good idea to order an X-ray and a urine analysis. It seems obvious to me now. It was a humiliating experience that prompted some soul searching. I asked myself, what does it mean to be a real doctor? And the answer came: a real doctor is someone who can handle an emergency. So, I went back and took training in emergency medicine, where you learn to ferret out problems that are really problems."

The next seven chapters consist mainly of excerpts from our 250 interviews, organized into categories of healing practices. Together, they constitute a portrait of an important aspect of private practice, in which doctors employ methods they acquired subsequent to their formal training. These chapters will acquaint you with a variety of unconventional treatments, as physicians explain how they discovered them, when and why they use them, and what their results have been. Needless to say, these treatments should be used only when approved and monitored by a physician. In the next two chapters we focus on the conceptual shift that has been instrumental in transforming modern medicine: the vanishing boundaries between mind and body.

CHAPTER 2

RECOGNIZING THE
POWER OF THE MIND

At the time I completed my medical training, psychiatrists were treated as the poor cousins of "real doctors." They were often seen as well-meaning people who somehow went wrong when choosing their specialties. Occasionally, if a patient acted crazy, the psychiatrists might be called in, but for the most part, their role was limited to treating the classical mental and emotional disorders. The role of psychoanalysts was mainly to treat neuroses and personality problems. At clinical meetings where "real illnesses" were discussed, the opinions of psychiatrists were solicited in the obligatory manner and politely endured, but our ideas usually fell on deaf ears. One famous physician at the time summed up the general attitude: "Psychiatrists disdain facts and worship words."

We have come a long way since then. The dichotomy between emotional states and somatic conditions has gradually broken down. In addition to our greater understanding of psychosomatic illness, we now accept *somatopsychic* illness. Classic mental disorders such as bipolar depression and the schizophrenias are now considered to have biological origins, just as physical disorders may be caused or exacerbated by severe emotional disturbances such as excessive anger, chronic anxiety, or fear. We are now at the point where it makes sense to postulate a single functional unit of psychophysiology, what some have termed "body-mind."

In addition, scientific evidence is mounting in support of an observation as old as medicine: the patient's attitude plays a significant role in determining the outcome of disease. In one study of women who had mastectomies, for example, those who had "fighting spirit" were twice as likely to be alive and well ten years after surgery than those with a hopeless, helpless attitude. Early evidence suggests that the mind has a direct effect on the body's ability to resist disease through its influence on the immune system.

It is, therefore, not surprising that when we asked doctors how their practices have changed since they completed their formal training, the most frequent responses had to do with the importance of psychology. Even the most orthodox physicians said that they have come to appreciate the significance of the mind and emotions in the prevention and treatment of disease. The more conservative doctors might merely advise patients to manage stress more effectively by changing their lifestyles or refer an emotionally disturbed patient to a psychiatrist. Others actually practice some form of psychotherapy themselves, using commonsense counseling methods or techniques acquired through private study or personal experience. A vocal minority contend that thoughts and feelings influence physical conditions to a far greater extent than mainstream medicine is prepared to accept. These doctors tend to emphasize psychological factors in diagnosing and treating illness, and to employ unusual therapeutic techniques.

One point on which there was notable unanimity concerned the need to spend more time getting to know patients and their families. This rather old-fashioned notion may be a reaction to the current dominance of pharmaceuticals and impersonal high-tech procedures. The doctors' comments imply that medicine is still largely an art and that the proper focus should be the individual patient, not the disease as such. They rejected the assumption that all patients with the same disorder can be treated the same way.

Several doctors noted that taking time to understand a patient's thoughts, feelings, and social milieu runs counter to another trend: cost-effective medicine. "It might sound crude to compare a sick person to a retail customer," said one, "but you don't need an MBA to figure out that the more patients you can see in the course of a day, the more revenue you can generate. Insurance companies and governments reimburse according to diagnosis, not the amount of time you spend with patients." Hence, if someone has, say, migraine headaches, it is more cost-effective to write a prescription than to explore how his history, relationships, or lifestyle affects the condition. Our interviews suggest that, despite the financial disincentive, some doctors are reaffirming the medical value of personal involvement.

It will be some time before we know exactly how, and to what extent, the mind can harm or heal the body. And it is too early to know the exact ways to instill in patients those attitudes that advance the healing process. The majority of physicians still feel ill-equipped by training and temperament to take on the role of psychotherapist. This will no doubt change as we learn more about the mind-body relationship, and as doctors realize that it now behooves them to add psychological training to their repertoire in order to provide optimal care. Among other things, our interviews point to a future where the distinction between healers of the mind and healers of the body will no longer be relevant.

In the first group of excerpts, doctors speak in general terms about the importance of psychological issues. Here is a family doctor in the Midwest: "I think the weakness of medical training is how to approach the mind—at least it was that way when I was in school. We talked some about it, but it wasn't pragmatic—all lecture and no lab—like how to sit down with patients and openly discuss their emotional conflicts. When I was a resident, a portion of our time was spent learning some basic interview techniques, but it was poorly developed. A lot of it was trial and error. I've had to teach myself from experience. Every day I spend time talking with people about life problems, ranging from job and marital difficulties to depression and stress management. I do some of it myself, and I actively refer to mental health professionals.

"For example, I frequently see patients with abdominal pain, and I end up talking about how they adapt to the pressures of work, home, and family. I'm dealing now with a twenty-two-year-old who has abdominal pain syndrome that's clearly related to his inability to cope and having to live at home with his parents. In children it's called Recurrent Abdominal Pains—stomach aches due to a nonorganic cause. I work with the parents to find the source of the child's anxiety. Often the children are perfectionists or high-achievers, and their expectations, or their parents' expectations, are disproportionate to performance. Under these circumstances it is necessary to help them achieve more realistic expectation levels.

"Headaches are another recurring problem. It's a challenge for patients to consider that some head pain may be a maladaptive response to stress, and that the use of medication is only palliative. It would be best to either reduce the stress or find more appropriate adaptive behaviors."

The next doctor, a family physician and professor at an East Coast medical school, addressed the overuse of high-tech diagnostic procedures at the expense of personal contact. "This trend is the result of two forces: the replacement of family doctors by emergency rooms and clinics, and the outbreak of malpractice suits, which have forced doctors to practice defensive medicine to rule out all diagnostic possibilities.

"Right out of training, I tried to solve every problem with specific tests, no matter what the expense, inconvenience, or risk. But, over time, I began to focus on the patient's story and our personal contact to better understand what was going on. This doesn't imply a distrust of testing procedures, but a healthier appreciation of their limitations. I would much rather tell a patient to call me back as soon as he feels something is changing than to run a test right away. I now keep more closely in touch with my patients. A physician who has continuity of care can do that. Somebody who is hospital-based never sees his patients after they are discharged.

"I wouldn't deny testing, but many of the tests available at tertiary care hospitals are extremely expensive and have high false-positive rates, and the wrong test can lead to inappropriate treatment. There is no better test than careful, watchful waiting, provided that a reasonable diagnosis safely allows you a little bit of time. If your diagnosis is one that compels you to act quickly, then that's what you have to do.

"I can give you many examples. I am seeing an eleven-year-old girl who suffers with severe headaches. The kid is bright and articulate, with a theatrical flair. If she were seen by emergency room physicians who don't know anything about her, she might get a CAT scan, an MRI, an EEG, and a lot of other expensive tests.

"But, the kid is from a family that's undergoing an acrimonious divorce. She started to develop headaches at the time the ugly confrontations surfaced, and she discovered that one way to keep her parents from tearing each other apart was to divert them with her symptoms. She can't articulate that, but she's learned that the way to diffuse painful interpersonal stresses is to get sick. And so, anytime there is conflict between the parents, she gets a headache.

"If she ends up in the emergency room, they give her a bunch of tests. On the other hand, I am aware of her difficulties and know the family history of migraine headache. Generally I would do a neurological and complete physical exams. If I don't see any markers for tumors or seizure disorder or vascular problems, I will try to clarify the psychodynamics behind the headache.

"The treatment is supportive psychotherapy. The best way to prevent these somatic responses from becoming ingrained is to help the parents see how their behavior affects their child. Obviously, you can't do that in the emergency room. However, if a kid is acting sick, and it's a scary headache, and you don't have any other alternatives, you tend to order a lot of tests and are more likely to prescribe major pain medications."

An anesthesiologist who runs a multidisciplinary pain clinic in Los Angeles had recently added a psychologist to his team. He said, only half joking: "I tell my psychologist that I keep the patients entertained and busy while she cures them. I call it integrated therapy. You can't just treat a part of someone. You have to treat the whole person or it doesn't work.

"Maybe I'm successful because I get the patients to acknowledge that there's an emotional component to their pain. Seventy-five percent of the patients we treat have stress-related problems. They are depressed, ache all over, have upset stomachs, and their posture has gone to pot. Ulcers and tension headaches don't always have a physical origin."

The next physician works in a community health center in New England. She began to change her approach when she became aware of a connection between certain physical complaints and specific traumatic events in her patients' past: "At some point, I realized that several young women whom I had attended for various medical problems—contraception, pelvic and abdominal pain—had histories of attempted suicides. When I got to know them better, I learned that they had all been sexually abused. Since that revelation, whenever I see a depressed young woman, I routinely ask about sexual abuse. Unfortunately, I'm beginning to find that this is all too common. It certainly affects my choice of treatment. For example, I have a thirteen-year-old patient who gets terrible headaches. Ordinarily, I might worry that she has some vascular disorder or a tumor. But I learned that she became pregnant a year ago—the result of being molested by her grandfather. This history influences my judgment as to what further lab tests or referrals are necessary.

"Knowing about past traumas can also be critical in discussing certain management issues. For instance, some women refuse to have a Pap smear. This is sometimes related to their having been sexually violated in the past. If I can discuss that openly with them, it can make all the difference."

This Los Angeles general practitioner said that he learned over time how important it was to listen closely to his patients: "What they *say* they've come to you for is often not what they really want. I've learned to listen with a third ear to find out what's really going on. The best time is when the patient is walking out the door: 'By the way, Doc, could my headaches be affecting my sex life?' Or sometimes it's, 'You know, I have this *friend*...' That's what you have to tune in to, beyond the obvious symptom."

He added: "The thing that's most effective with patients is to give them a sense of caring about themselves. I spend a great deal of time talking to people with hypertension, migraines, tension headaches, and many physical problems with an emotional overlay. I try to impress upon them that they have to like themselves. They have to change their emotional environments. I try to affirm that they're worthwhile human beings who deserve to feel good and live long lives. Sometimes I scare my patients, particularly those with hypertension. I show them morbidity tables, I tell them if they don't take care of themselves they might live, but they'll be crippled. They'll have impaired kidney function, strokes, circulatory problems, and memory loss. Then I say, 'When you're ready for help, we'll do this together.' It's always 'we'—the patient and me. Letting them know you care is three quarters of the battle. They want to know that they're not just another number to you, not just another fee. I began to really understand the significance of that in my later years in practice."

A rural practitioner in Northern California cites obese patients as examples of when psychological savvy is needed: "I have men and women who are double their ideal body weight with no physical cause. They suffer terrible disability. Many have resorted to gastric bypasses and other high-tech or surgical solutions, which in my experience have not been successful. They're just incredibly troubled. It's not that they don't know what they're supposed to be eating. Clearly they're not eating out of hunger. There are lots of reasons for that particular form of gluttony. They're hiding out, not dealing with issues that food is the cover-up for. They usually have traumatic histories that you learn about in time, about how unhappy and mistreated they were as kids. Sometimes I get them to open up, sometimes not at all.

"One lady I'm dealing with now weighs 286 and she's only about five feet four. She's taking large doses of antidepressants from the county mental health facility. She's a heavy user of alcohol and drugs. I also met her divorced mother. I didn't like her. She was taking Valium and always complaining about her boyfriend. All of a sudden, it struck me how devoted my patient was to her mother. I talked to her about it, and this story emerged. As a child, she had been abused by a couple of the mother's boyfriends, and the mother knew it was going on and did nothing about it."

The doctor said he helped his patient see the connection between her early abuse and her gluttony. "She's able to talk more freely about her past and is starting to lose weight and stay sober. Her eating habits are still abnormal, but she's improving. The problem I have as an internist is that I become so involved with patients that I wish I were a psychiatrist."

Finally, a cardiologist describes the experience that convinced him, early in his career, to add psychotherapeutic procedures to his practice: "I was working with people who had been to the best cardiovascular centers in America and had every procedure known to man. Nothing was left. So I would sit and talk to them. I discovered that they got angina when they fought with their spouse or when their children upset them. I found this so interesting that I'd ask them more, and they'd say, 'Aren't you a cardiologist? Why do you want to know about my wife, or whether I'm happy at work?' Well, because those were the precipitating events for the angina.

"One woman had four major drugs to reduce blood pressure, and it was still elevated. During the interview, I asked her how many children she had. She said hesitantly, 'Two . . . one.' And I caught it.

I went on with the interview, and at the end, after examining her, I asked her, 'I'm not clear. How many children did you say you have?' And she started crying. She said, 'I've never talked to anyone about this. It happened six years ago.'

"I asked her when the hypertension began. 'Six years ago.' It turned out her son had been killed in an auto accident back then. She loved him and had told him not to go out that night. She ended up blaming herself all that time and had kept it inside. Once she made the breakthrough, she didn't have that bottled-up pressure of denial."

THE DOCTOR-PATIENT BOND

Many of our respondents spoke of the importance of a close doctor-patient relationship. They felt this helped to inspire trust and faith, which they believe is a powerful but undervalued component of healing. They were convinced that a good, caring relationship can shorten recovery time. First, a woman who has been practicing since 1955:

"Those things that make up bedside manner: gestures, facial expressions, tone of voice, almost anything done in a caring way, are very important. Patients who have confidence in me often say that they start getting well in the waiting room or on their way here.

"It's a mysterious relationship. Getting sick is a mystery, and getting well is twice the mystery. The attitude of the doctor also plays an important role in the recovery process. If the doctor's an s.o.b. whose mannerisms say, 'Don't bother me, take this, lotsa luck!' he is cheating the patient."

An internist who has been in practice nearly thirty years believes that the doctor-patient bond strengthens the power of suggestion: "There has to be a combination of strong expectation by the patient and great belief by the doctor. With that combination of an enthusiastic therapist and a receptive patient you'll often get this extraordinary effect of a heightened power of suggestion. If we had a way of effectively using this, we would save a lot of penicillin. I've had patients say that they got better because they didn't want to hurt me, or they knew how upset I'd be if they didn't get better."

The same doctor said he tries to involve patients in making decisions, both because he trusts their intuition and because it strengthens their commitment to the treatment process: "I see patients an average of a half hour per visit, so there's time to establish a relationship. My feeling is that if my recommendation doesn't make sense to them, then there is a high probability that something is wrong. If they don't understand it, then we have to spend more time until we mutually agree."

A veteran internist with positions at a major metropolitan hospital and medical school said he tries to foster what he considers the right attitude in his patients: "I have never used any unorthodox treatments other than affirmative thinking. I always say you have nothing to lose by encouraging strong, positive thoughts, and you have everything in the world to lose by being a pessimist. Patients who are optimists are easier to manage. They get better faster, and if they *don't,* they at least survive their illness with fewer complications.

"I give pep talks. If I have a bad diagnosis to deliver I always tell the truth, but I always start with the positive aspects of the particular disease. There are plenty of negative ones, but you don't have to lead with them. For example, if a cancer patient complains about problems associated with the illness, I will never say, 'The reason you're having this is because of the cancer.' I will say, 'The reason you're having this is because you're getting heartburn or indigestion, perhaps something you ate.' I'm practicing what we call 'denial.' It's a very good defense mechanism, which often helps. If I tell them, 'You're having your symptoms because of the cancer or the chemotherapy,' that would work against what I'm trying to accomplish. I would say, 'You're having indigestion, we have a treatment for it, and this is what we're going to do.' I never bring up the bogey man again. If they say, 'Is this because of chemotherapy?' I say, 'That might be, but it's also a possibility that it's something you ate.'

"I won't fib knowingly, but I don't want them to accept hopeless-ness. I have to give them a little thread to hang on to. With a diagnosis of lupus I would say, 'Have you heard of the term arthritis?' If they say, 'Yes,' I reply, 'Well, this is like an arthritis of all the connective tissue of the body, which can produce all kinds of symptoms, for example: achiness, skin rash, and kidney problems.' Now, they've heard of arthritis a million times, and they know it doesn't kill anybody. That analogy is apt because lupus is a connective tissue disorder that involves other areas besides the joints, and we treat it the same way, with anti-inflammatory medicine."

Interestingly, the same doctor told us that he sometimes deliber-ately uses placebos with his patients, a surprising admission from someone who considers himself mainstream. Placebos are now re-garded as mere adjuncts to research; inert substances used as controls when testing the efficacy of an actual medication. But the repeated observation that patients might actually improve when unknowingly given placebos has led many researchers to ponder how a positive mind-set can produce real physical changes. In one study, a placebo was dispensed by a machine to a group of patients who were told that it was pain medication. A second group was given the same substance by a physician in a white coat with a stethoscope in his pocket and a big syringe. Not surprisingly, the patients who were given the placebo by a confidence-inspiring doctor reported much less pain.

That same internist told us this story: "A patient came to me with arthritis. She had been seeing a doctor who'd been administering cortisone injections and prescribing various drugs, which had not been very helpful. We were seeing bad effects from the medication, and, if anything, the arthritis was getting worse. Nevertheless, this was giving her momentary relief.

"Well, I felt the temporary relief of cortisone was not worth the side effects of long-term use, like joint degeneration. I got to know this patient. She liked and respected me, and she knew I was trying to help her. I would tell her I was giving her an injection of cortisone, but I was actually using a placebo because the cortisone was hurting her. A little belt of saline solution in her buttock gave her three or four days of relief, just as if it had been cortisone and without any side effects.

"In my twenty-seven years of practice I've done this maybe a dozen times, mostly with addicts. For example, take patients who are addicted to Percodan. I might recognize that it is not doing them a damn bit of good anymore, that they're habituated to it, and it's giving them devastating side effects. But I can't switch to anything else. They know the color of the pill, and they want it. So I go to the hospital pharmacy and say, 'Make me a pill that looks like Percodan.' They'd give me an antihistamine or something, and in the dark room, a patient who's getting two pills every four hours and is more or less comfortable won't know the difference. After a while, he's not taking Percodan, but two pills that *looked* like Percodan but are safer and can be controlled easily."

No one quite knows how placebos work. The most commonly held theory is that the brain might release endorphins (natural pain-reducing substances that mimic the structure of opiates) not only when a person is in pain but when he believes he's been given pain medication. Regardless of the mechanisms involved, the mere fact that placebos can improve a patient's condition has convinced many doctors that faith, trust, and positive thinking have healing powers.

A gynecologist comments on the importance of the patient's faith in the physician, especially when treatment entails deprivation and pain: "I doubt that anything can be accomplished unless there is a transference of faith between doctor and patient. When it's present, there's a sense of power—just the physical presence of the physician makes that person feel better. I've had patients tell me that by just walking in the office they felt better. For example, there is a thirty-eight-year-old lady who came to see me regarding a pelvic mass. Before I actually did the diagnostic surgery, I suspected that we were dealing with cancer. And, in fact, it turned out to be a very advanced malignancy.

"I have a very aggressive approach toward cancer. I don't just take a little biopsy but try to excise all the cancer tissue. In this case, I was able to remove everything with the exception of the right kidney. There was no way I could get it without removing the kidney, and it still wouldn't have helped because the whole area was rampant with the spread of ovarian cancer. According to the textbooks, she should have been dead within eighteen months.

"Following surgery, I started her on chemotherapy right away. I explained that I use chemotherapy a little differently in that I push the dosage beyond its recommended levels. There may be serious complications in doing that, but I want to cure patients, not just prolong their life an extra six months. She got awfully sick, but she stayed on chemo for eighteen months. The point is, she had to have great faith in me to consent to that radical procedure, but she's been tumor-free for seven years now. She has a full life that's not compromised on any level.

"During the process, I recommend psychotherapy. I do this with all cancer patients. I sent her to an excellent psychiatrist, and she terminated after six months because she felt so convinced I was going to cure her that she didn't have to prepare for death."

The physician also made a point of warning against putting *too* much faith in faith. "I think that confidence and a positive attitude are of tremendous importance, and yet we see people who exemplify those attributes but don't beat their illness. Then there are those who *don't* have those beliefs and go into remission anyway. So, you wonder. I've seen fantastic people whom I've really loved, respected, and admired, who gave it their all, but couldn't do anything to even improve their illnesses. I think it is correlated with the individual's immune system and connections with those levels of consciousness that we don't completely understand."

A Santa Monica practitioner, known for an eclectic repertoire and informal relations with patients, described his basic approach: "A lot of what I do is just talk with people. My goal is to really know my patients, know how they think, know the way they are, know their character, so that when they're *out* of character I know it. I take a long history. I ask a lot of pretty intense questions. I want to know, does their life work? I like patient participation. Many patients go to a doctor and they say the doctor healed them, but the patient allowed it!"

When we interviewed a cardiologist, we noted that his office was as casual as a living room. He explained: "I always think back to my family physician. He was very loving and caring, and I modeled myself after him. One of the doctors who refers people to me calls me a 'non-white-coat doctor.' Some people would rather see me with a white coat, stethoscope, and tie. When they walk into this office, I can see it in their faces. I don't admit anyone to my practice if I don't feel some rapport. This is determined by the initial interview. If I feel an incompatibility, I share that with them. If I don't think we'd be a good match, I refer them to someone else. My work has a lot to do with the patient feeling safe. I think one of the best folk remedies is love. The heart is not just a pump. Cardiac disorders can have something to do with disharmony on the level of giving and receiving love."

The next physician, a general practitioner in Malibu, agrees that love is, indeed, an important component of healing: "In my heart, I believe I love people to health. I think my willingness to love and accept them helps patients to love and accept themselves. And that's healing. I mainly talk with people and listen to them. Most of my first appointments are an hour long because people often come with complex problems. I try to get an understanding of who's sitting across from me, and I try to help *them* hear what they're actually saying.

"After that initial appointment, the first thing I do with most people is a basic medical workup, physical exam, blood tests, and allergy tests if necessary. There are many ways that a person is healed. There's not just one answer. We have to find what fits. Part of my original intake is learning what will work for them, and I start there.

"Once we initiate a common understanding, and they feel safe, then

I can move to a deeper level. I work on helping people to love themselves, and to see that the way they feel about themselves really affects their body. I have mirrors in my office, and sometimes I'll ask people to stand up and look in the mirror. Not look at their eyes, or their hands, or their hips, or their hair, but to look at the whole person for a while, and then tell that person that they love him or her. I can remember the most dramatic instance, a lady who had been hospitalized with clinical depression and whom I had told to do this exercise. One day she informed me that she had not been able to do it. She would say it, but she didn't mean it. So I stood her up in front of the mirror, and she looked in the mirror, and she wouldn't do it. She absolutely refused. So I said the words with her, and I held her while she said it. She just melted and turned into a little child. And I asked her to take the time to do it every day and learn to mean it. It turned the course of her healing around. The program she was on had a much better chance to work."

UNUSUAL THERAPIES

While most of the doctors confine their involvement in patient psychology to informal counseling, a number have acquired therapeutic techniques through independent study. Some told us about their use of unusual forms of psychotherapy. Here is an example—a cardiologist who uses a technique called *voice dialogue:*

"When I tried to refer some of my cardiac patients to a therapist, they would balk. They wanted me to do it. I started to do some counseling, but I wanted something that wasn't so time-consuming. I asked around, and someone sent me to Dr. Harold Stone, who was working with cancer patients. I trained with him and incorporated his technique of voice dialogue into my work. It involves getting patients in touch with their feelings and thoughts about their illness."

Voice dialogue assumes that each individual is made up of various "sub-personalities" that represent different attributes. The physician explained: "The procedure allows the person to adopt a sub-personality, which I can then communicate with. For example, I might tell a patient to move into another chair because I want to talk to the part of him that is angry. And that part comes out and says, essentially, 'Hello, what do you want?' 'I want to know a little about you. Who are you? How did you get this way? How do you influence his health?'

"And I get responses like these: 'I get him good. If he's at a party, I make him eat all the cheese. I know his cholesterol is high.' Or I speak to the sub-personality that's angry, and it might say something like, 'He ignores me. He's always working, so I get angry and give him chest pain.' " According to the physician, the information that comes up during the dialogue can lead to further discussion and eventually a change in behavior. "The patients have to be aware that negative thoughts and feelings cause physical changes that can affect their health. I work with them to get them to see that."

He also uses the voice dialogue method to help reluctant patients comply with his recommendations. "Usually there is a lot of resistance, so I talk to the part that refuses to exercise. I hear, 'Boy, that scares me. What if I sprain my ankle? What if I have a heart attack?' And I learn they're afraid something bad will happen if they exercise. I have them use the treadmill while I'm there to reassure them. That conditions them positively, and they lose their fear of exercise."

A number of physicians said they integrate physical and psychological methods, sometimes turning to unorthodox approaches. Representative of that group is this Los Angeles psychiatrist: "I take a systems approach. I look at individuals as part of a larger context. They're living with a family, living in a community, a culture, living in a physical environment that might be toxic. And the individuals themselves are also systems of mind, body, and spirit. I try to address all of that when evaluating which treatment will be most effective."

As an example, she spoke of patients with chronic fatigue syndrome, the number of whom, she says, has increased in recent years. "Their antibody levels are usually pretty high. I treat them with special diets in addition to psychotherapy because the immune system is very much affected by mood states. Depression definitely causes suppression of T-cells. There's no question that if you alleviate depression, the immune system will be stimulated and better able to deal with these viruses, which may be secondary to a depressed immune system rather than the opposite. I saw a woman who had allergies to practically everything. When she met a guy and started a relationship, her symptoms got much better, her antibody levels improved, and the amount of supplements she needed to feel normal went down. That really impressed me. It wasn't that she was faking before, but now she felt good about herself, she'd become sexually active—which she hadn't been in years—and was in this passionate relationship with a man who adored her. So she got better. Love really does heal. A lot of people who are ill don't love themselves. Sometimes they need somebody else. Being in love is really being in love within oneself, and that has a positive effect on the immune system."

With regard to the unorthodox techniques that she uses, she said, "Everything I do I've picked up; it didn't come with my original education. My psychiatric training was psychoanalytic, but I saw that as pretty limited. It's probably useful as a model of how the unconscious might work, but it didn't give me the tools to heal people. I found that I was more comfortable with a more humanistic therapeutic approach than with the traditional school of psychoanalysis. Psychotherapy has more to offer than it used to, such as guided imagery, psychosynthesis, and neurolinguistic programming. What you really try to do in psychotherapy is to encourage catharsis. You uncover the old traumatic situation, get in touch with it, and relive it. But there are developing technologies where you not only relive a traumatic event but you can recreate the memory and replace it with new memories.

"One of my methods is called inner child work. It's getting people in touch with their early traumas. I've done some interesting things using an imagery scene of a traumatic childhood experience. I would then bring in the inner good parent to comfort the child and explain to him that it wasn't his fault, that he's really a wonderful, loveable child, and that the parent was going to be with him forever. In doing that, you're installing good parenting, so the inner child has someone who loves it, and in turn can feel loveable. The next step is using the imagery techniques to literally refashion the memory. It changes the substrate of how you're feeling and thinking in such a way that the patient begins to feel better about himself.

"I treated a man who recalled an incestuous experience with his father. I not only had him go through the scene, but then had his adult self confront his father and say, 'I want you to know what impact this has had on me—and what happened the rest of my life as a result of your behavior.' In the scene, his father cried and was very remorseful. Then I had the patient create scenes of childhood in which his father was a *good* father, where they played ball together and did all those things he'd actually wanted his father to do but had never done. The result was that he started to do better. He said, 'I don't know what's going on. Things are just going better for me. I'm not trying to do anything differently. It's just happening.' "

The following excerpt is from a Los Angeles physician who treats patients with a mixture of unorthodox methods, both physical and mental. "One guy came here just absolutely panic-stricken. In these cases, I usually ask the patients to do abdominal breathing many times during the day. This helps to diminish their fears. But he had chronic nasal stuffiness. It was one of those times where a voice went off in my head and said, 'He needs a complete workup.' So I told him, 'Just so I can sleep at night, I want you to get such and such tests done.' Diagnostic testing is one of the areas in which American medicine shines. It turned out he had a non-operable lymphoma. I advised him to go home and deal with his family and take care of business. I truly believed in my heart that he had about four months to live.

"I also had him do visualization exercises. I don't like the kind where you visualize armies eating up these horrible little invaders. It can work, but I think people get further by doing something calm and gentle, so I asked him to visualize a lot of white light gently dissolving the tumor. I led him through the steps and had him go home and do it himself. He came back and said, 'I feel so different. I feel so at peace with this.' In the next several months all his X-rays and biopsies came back negative. They discounted it as a spontaneous remission: 'It just happened to go away, and we don't know why.' Every time he goes back to his ENT specialist, they pull out dead cells. He's amazing. I've had other patients echo the same themes."

The same physician specializes in treating AIDS with unconventional approaches. "The patients who do best are the ones who look at the AIDS virus as their friend. I tell them to read the book by Will N. George, *Beyond AIDS,* which is a chronicle of what two people have done to deal with this illness. It talks about empowerment and about loving your cells, including the part called the AIDS virus; it also talks about how fear can disrupt the immune system. Anything they can do to diminish their fear is going to help them enhance their positive response.

"My star patient of all time was one of those whose spirit enabled him to live a longer and fuller life than his prognosis would have predicted. He was so feisty and earthy and authentic. He'd had Kaposi's sarcoma when I saw him. He was stable, but was drifting downward, and he wanted some advice. I told him he should stop smoking, and he threw his cigarettes away, and that was the end of it. When you get people who are willing to participate, it's thrilling. He went on herbal medicine and started doing his own research and checking out everything. His diarrhea and weight loss stopped. His energy increased. He continued along, working full-time, jogging every day, in good health. He had no deterioration for years. When he finally died, he was tumor-free."

In our next excerpt, a Southern California doctor speaks of her research with cancer patients. "We were operating under the notion that if cancer patients could become more aware, they could help their immune system become strengthened and improved. We had observed that cancer patients tended to be too nice—the type of people who kept a lot of their feelings in. People who yell a lot get high blood pressure or heart attacks or strokes, but nice people who accepted their fate and didn't fight too much got cancer. About ten percent of the people who get cancer say, 'Hey, I'm not going to stand for this. I want to do something about it.' Those were the people we worked with—the fighters.

"We did high-intensity confrontation groups where people would really get their feelings out. We tried to discover reasons why they permitted their immune systems to fail and why they might have lost their will to live. We uncovered a lot of interesting trends. Many of the patients were holding in feelings that needed to get out, like anger and pain. One woman had a really bad marriage and was financially dependent. She felt trapped and helpless. We saw this often, and the ones who had the courage to confront the problem improved the quality of their lives tremendously. With impending death as a motive to change their lives, people become more alive and more aware. This is why some people say that although cancer is terrible, it has also given them a valuable lesson. Many lives were prolonged.

"Our doctors never interfered with the healing work that the patients were doing. The oncologists would come and talk to the patients. Of course, some of them saw us as a threat and *didn't* visit, but some of them were wonderful, and the patients they sent us came with a totally different attitude. They were positive, and they looked at chemotherapy as an ally to their own inner resources for helping their immune systems, not as a poison that was going to work against them. Occasionally, we would get people who insisted that they were going to do it themselves and *not* get chemotherapy. We discouraged that. The body lags behind the psyche. Your psyche might be totally healed, but the body takes three to six months, and you need the chemotherapy to maintain you while you get your immune system in balance. Most of the people, by the time they came to us, had already had chemotherapy, surgery, radiation, the whole bit, and more or less said, 'Well, whatever you can do, go ahead.'

"With seriously ill patients," the doctor added, "the goal of psycho-therapeutic intervention is not necessarily to cure but to comfort and facilitate the growth of understanding. When we started out, our egos were involved: 'We're going to save these people. We're going to cure them.' We realized we were also involved with improving the quality of life: how to get in touch with your feelings, how to let people know that you love them and help them to live a better life. That was the most important contribution. One patient I remember well, a man with cancer of the bladder. He was indomitable in terms of the will to survive and fight. He loved the work. He lasted for eleven years. When he finally got one of his last recurrences, my ego was saying, 'You've got to keep fighting. You can't let up.' He said he didn't want to disappoint me, but he asked me to let him go. It was an incredible lesson. I realized that people have the right to give up the fight. He had fought hard for eleven years. When he died, he was a more profound person, a more conscious person, and he had a much deeper appreciation of life."

REMARKABLE HEALING

We close this chapter with stories of remarkable recoveries that our respondents attributed to psychological factors. The first is from a psychiatrist who is frequently sent patients by other specialists who want to supplement their treatments with psychotherapy: "I recall one patient who had an ulcer that would periodically bleed and was not responding to medical treatment. He was reluctant to have surgery. He was afraid and was sure it would mean certain death. For this reason, the surgeon had postponed recommending an operation for years, but he got to the point where he felt it was vital. So he sent the patient to me to help him overcome his fear of surgery. Well, in the process of working with him, I uncovered the sources of tension that were contributing to his ulcer. Ultimately, he not only overcame his fear of surgery and agreed to have the operation, but he said, 'You know, I've been feeling so much better, I haven't had any trouble with my stomach.' So I sent him back to the surgeon, and they took another X-ray, and the ulcer had healed. The surgeon said, 'I'm never going to send a patient to you again.'

"So, you sometimes see incredible results. My concept is that the subconscious mind has a powerful influence on our capacity to get well. The patient's convictions, his own beliefs, are extremely important. I did work at one time with the Navajo Indians. There was a medicine man on the hospital staff. He would chant and do the sand painting ceremony—which has great significance to the Indians—and that would sometimes do them more good than our conventional medicines."

In the next story, a physician gave more of herself than would normally be expected, with what proved to be dramatic results. The following experience influenced the way she would subsequently approach her patients. "I was a resident doing a pediatrics rotation, and I admitted a sixteen-year-old girl with myasthenia gravis [a debilitating auto-immune disease characterized by muscular weakness]. She was having a relapse. She was a beautiful, sad girl, really pitiful, and I looked at her and asked, 'Why is this happening to you?' The next morning, when I went to make rounds, she was sort of cheery. She said, 'Will you come back and talk to me after work? I've been talking to my roommate, who said I should tell you everything.'

"Well, she related the most horrible story of the crazy, sick family she was raised in and of being sexually abused by all of her father's friends. She said that the only time she got her family to quiet down and for the craziness to stop was when she got sick. She was suicidal because of what she had to go through. I think making the connection between her illness and her molestation had a big impact on her. She connected with someone who cared. I became like her big sister and helped her get out of that house and find other resources. She went into therapy. She still had plenty of pain and suffering to go through, but she had unlocked the door. Fortunately, from that moment on, she never had another myasthenia attack. The last I heard, she was a happily married woman."

Then there is this account by an internist who specializes in immunology: "About twenty years ago, I was called in to see a woman who was supposed to have brain surgery the next day. All they asked me to do was check out her heart. So I did, and everything was okay, but I thought I'd just get into the neurological part, which I was not asked to do. The woman had gradually lost the ability to use one side of her body. I gave her a little barbiturate intravenously—enough to make her just a little woozy—and I started talking to her about events at the time the problem started. I found that she had seen her father for the first time in fifteen years, and she'd felt guilty about the way in which they'd split. From that point on, her left leg had begun to get numb and weak. So I borrowed a pin from the nurse, who was standing there, and I pushed it into this woman's hand on the paralyzed side. She pulled it back. I pricked the sole of her foot. She pulled it back. She could feel it. When she woke up, she was paralyzed again. I had called her doctor and told him about it, and he canceled the surgery. It took a week of psychotherapy, and she was okay. I feel that it might have saved her life."

By way of injecting some humor into his interview, and to make a point about not leaping to conclusions in the face of unusual recoveries, the same internist recalled another event: "I was called one Sunday to see a patient in the hospital. I was just out of my residency, and the nurse was very frank. She said I was the sixth internist they called and they couldn't get any of their first five choices. So I went to the hospital, and when I walked into the room, I saw an old lady lying there. They said she'd been unconscious for two days. I put my mouth down to her ear and I yelled, "Wake up!" And she jumped right up. Just then, the head nurse opened the door and saw me holding this lady, and she ran down the hall yelling, 'A miracle! A miracle!' Well,

I moved from number-six internist to number-one. And you know what I think it was? This was an old lady who got disoriented and scared. She was hard of hearing, and she just laid down still, closed her eyes, and didn't want to know what was going on. She was fine after that and went home."

Our interviews suggest that doctors are increasingly aware of how the mind can make the body sick as well as how it can help make it well. Naturally, if that is true, it stands to reason that the reverse might also be true: physical factors have an impact on the mind and emotions. In the next chapter, we consider that side of the mind-body coin.

CHAPTER 3

DISCOVERING THE PHYSICAL
SIDE OF MENTAL HEALTH

W hen mental disorders were first classified by terms such as hysteria, dementia, and mania, it was natural that the search for causes would center on psychological processes such as unresolved mental conflicts, developmental traumas, and inappropriate defense mechanisms. From there, it was a short step to declare that they should be treated in kind, through primarily psychological intervention. However, there were always dissenters who pointed out that while the symptoms of certain mental disorders seemed to center on cognitive and emotional abnormalities, we should continue the search for a physical etiology. They advocated looking to the brain for causes and treatments. Despite careful investigation, however, no one was able to find a confirmable organic basis for so-called functional mental disorders. Hence, the majority of mental health professionals concluded that psychological problems have psychological roots and should be treated in kind.

When it was seen that biochemical events in the body could strongly influence behavior, the brain-mind issue was revitalized and a vast new range of therapeutic possibilities opened up. From the 1940s on, drugs such as the antipsychotics, the antidepressants, and

Lithium began to be used widely to treat psychiatric disorders. A breakthrough occurred when researchers found correlations between substances found in the nervous system, known as neurotransmitters, and mental/emotional phenomena. This ultimately led to disagreement between the analytically oriented psychiatrists and those who favored pharmacological treatment. The former saw the pharmacological approach as ameliorative rather than curative. Additionally, it posed an existential dilemma: if behavior were indeed reducible to biochemistry, would life be robbed of free will and all the ethical and moral attributes we regard as uniquely human? When, in the 1980s, it was discovered that even obsessive-compulsive disorders yielded to pharmaceutical treatment, and when genetic links to certain mental conditions were established, it was no longer possible to deny the effective role of physical modalities in the treatment of psychological disorders.

By now, psychoactive drugs are standard treatment for depression, schizophrenia, and other diseases. However, in our interviews, we found that many physicians, psychiatrists for the most part, were less than fully satisfied with these medications. Some turned to unconventional biochemical approaches, mostly centering around nutrition. The excerpts we selected address that search for alternatives.

VITAMINS FOR THE MIND

A classically trained psychiatrist told us how his career was turned around by a colleague in the 1960s: "I was treating schizophrenics with medication and electroconvulsive therapy [ECT], but was dissatisfied with the results. I thought, 'There's got to be more to all the training I have had than ECT and Thorazine.' ECT, while effective in some very acute cases, often did not seem to have much lasting effect, and Thorazine kept people pretty much doped up. I was ripe for something. My hospital had about a thousand attending physicians, and I developed a working relationship with some of them.

"One of those physicians was an early proponent of orthomolecular psychiatry, which was then referred to as megavitamin therapy. Although I only spoke to him on the telephone and did not meet him for several months, I noticed that he prescribed large doses of vitamins. I thought, 'This is absolutely ridiculous. There can be nothing to this.' But, as long as he was continuing to use shock treatment, Thorazine, and the routine procedures, there was no objection.

"Then one day he called me and said, 'I have to leave town for about three weeks. Would you please cover for me?' I said, 'Covering for you is no problem, but I don't know what you're doing with your vitamins.' He said, 'I know you don't, but my patients know what they're supposed to do, and I just need you for patients who might require hospitalization.' During the next three weeks, I got some calls from families saying that the patient had either gone off the special diet or stopped the vitamins, and the symptoms had come back. This was something I hadn't seen with conventional medicine, so my interest was piqued.

"I said to myself, 'Either I can turn my back on this and continue to say it's just quackery, or I can look into it.' I had the time and opportunity, and it wasn't going to affect me economically one way or the other. I couldn't justify dismissing it. So I decided to observe his patients for six months. I found that his hospitalized patients were responding better than the others and that the megavitamin treatment seemed harmless. I adopted his regimen with my own patients.

"At the time, I had three schizophrenic patients who were either deteriorating or just barely functioning. I used to see them at least once a week. One girl would beg for shock treatment since it was the only thing that gave her any clarity, even if only for a few hours. I proposed adding megavitamin therapy to what we were doing, and all three were willing. After six or eight weeks, two of the three began to show some positive changes. The most striking was the girl who stopped her shock treatments and began to develop an interest in the other patients and her group activities. That was really exciting. They were all put on a low blood sugar diet with large doses of niacin or niacinamide, along with Vitamins C, B6, E, and other supportive vitamins, usually in addition to medication. I stayed at the hospital another couple of years and then went to work with the physician who introduced me to the new therapy."

Now, more than twenty years later, the psychiatrist has a private practice in Los Angeles, where he uses nutritional supplements and special diets to treat patients who would normally receive psychotherapy and drugs. Unorthodox veterans like him influenced some of the next generation of psychiatrists, one of whom told us:

"After my training, I found there were patients who weren't responding quickly enough to psychotherapy. I wanted to see if there was another approach. I began using orthomolecular techniques, which were not accepted in regular psychiatric circles. The more I got into it, the more I realized the importance of clinical nutrition and how much the endocrine system affects thoughts and moods. Not only can our minds cause illness, but physical illnesses can produce systemic imbalances that may lead to profound emotional and mental changes. Many people who come to me with psychiatric symptoms have *physical* problems, like allergies, viral infections, malnutrition, and endocrine disorders. Once we treat these conditions the psychological symptoms clear up."

These methods have become an essential part of her practice, especially with patients suffering from chronic depression, mood swings, and addiction withdrawal. "People will go to psychotherapists forever, and talk about their childhood and their problems, and I think that is useful. But everyone has stuff they can dig up. You can go over it ad nauseam, but a time comes when you have to look at something else. You may meet someone who's been in psychotherapy forever and hasn't had a breakthrough, and you check his diet and change it, and guess what? His mind clears up."

In many cases, she added, a physiological imbalance will affect the brain in such a way as to make it difficult for patients to respond to traditional talk therapy. "They can't think straight, their memory's gone, they can't concentrate, and it's hard for them to respond to psychotherapy. You can't do any real intensive psychotherapy until they're tracking better. At the same time, they need help dealing with friends and families who are telling them, 'There's nothing wrong with you. Get yourself out of this. Go out socially. Go back to your job.' This only intensifies their confusion and despair. So you have to carefully check their physical condition first."

She continues to prescribe traditional medicines, but does so sparingly: "Some people don't want to take a lot of vitamins, or they just don't do as well as they should with diet and supplements, so I'll use antidepressants. For some people, Prozac is a miracle drug; for others, it has side effects and doesn't work. The same is true for a lot of the supplements. I'll put someone on an amino acid, and he'll be wired; I'll put someone else on it, and he'll feel normal for the first time in his life. But the difference is not as marked as it is with the use of drugs. It's a more subtle physiological shift."

AMINO ACIDS AND MENTAL HEALTH

Amino acids are said to affect the mind and emotions because they are needed to manufacture neurotransmitters, the chemical messengers of the brain. For example, tryptophan, a precursor to the neurotransmitter serotonin, had been used with good effect with insomniacs until it was taken off the market after an outbreak of a rare muscular disorder was associated with its use. Other amino acids were mentioned by several of the doctors we interviewed. The comments of this Colorado internist were typical:

"People who are chronically stressed and are on a roller coaster of blood sugar going up and down are especially prone to dips in energy at certain times of day. Their adrenals are not functioning optimally, and when they hit a real low point, they want sugar. It usually happens in mid-afternoon when the adrenal glands are at their lowest level of functioning. I have them take glutamine at that point because it helps to regulate the glucose in the brain.

"I've also had good results with a naturally occurring substance called dimethylaminoethinol, or DMAE. For example, one of my female patients had been addicted to drugs but had been clean for about three years. She still complained of memory defects, and I suggested she try DMAE. It's a derivative of fish oil, but it happens to be a precursor to the neurotransmitter acetylcholine, which is implicated in memory processing. She tried it for a while, and her memory came back. It was really remarkable."

A number of psychiatrists and family doctors mentioned the amino acid tyrosine as an aid to treating ordinary depression and the emotional swings associated with premenstrual syndrome. Said one from the San Francisco Bay Area: "I've had great results with tyrosine. It's like a natural antidepressant and is a precursor to the neurotransmitter norepinephrine. Once the right dosage is determined, it usually works really well for people with mild depression or severe mood swings, especially if you add B vitamins."

It should be noted that most of the doctors who discussed amino acid and vitamin treatments declined to tell us the exact dosages they prescribe for specific conditions. Such determinations, they said, are best made on an individual basis, preferably with the help of blood or urine tests. However, some patients can't afford the lab work and not every insurance company will pay for it. In such cases, the Colorado internist said he prescribes conservatively and monitors the effect:

"I have them add one new supplement at a time and tell them to watch their body's reaction. If I suspect a food allergy, for example, I tell them to eliminate certain foods from their diet and later introduce them one at a time. It's like detective work. I had a woman who was heavily addicted to cocaine. She came to me quite depressed, and was not functioning very well at all. I assumed she was nutritionally depleted and put her on a really good multivitamin and mineral product and an assortment of amino acids. We kept adjusting her dosage and her diet, depending on what she experienced between visits, and gradually she was able to correct her own physiology. Within weeks she had a turnaround."

It is important to emphasize that there are degrees of individual difference in every person's response to therapy, and in some instances the range of reactions can be quite remarkable. It is the doctors' art to find these variances and tailor their treatment accordingly. The effects of a specific therapeutic agent may also change over time.

THE ELIMINATION OF SUGAR

A number of doctors spoke not of how they supplement their patients' diets, but of what they *eliminate* from them. Sugar and caffeine were singled out most often as troublemakers. Several physicians claimed that discontinuing the consumption of those substances can sometimes accomplish what years of psychotherapy cannot. Here is a New York-based general practitioner:

"I can give you many cases of people who came in with terrible mood swings, and I checked out their diet and eliminated Coke, coffee, and donuts, all those items that can result in severe blood sugar swings. The brain uses more glucose than any organ in the body, and glucose is a breakdown product of ordinary sugar. Certain people show chronic glucose deprivation. There's a sugar rush, then insulin is secreted, which brings the blood sugar way down. As a result, they can't think straight, they have emotional swings, anxiety, and tremors. If they went to most doctors, they would be treated with antidepressants or antianxiety agents. What I do is direct them toward correcting their diets.

"For example, a woman came in last month complaining that she was having extreme mood swings. She was fighting with her boyfriend, couldn't handle her work, and felt incredibly stressed in everything she did. Yet, her life, when you looked at it, wasn't externally stressful. Turns out she had been dieting, and she hadn't been able to lose weight although she'd kept her calories down, but she was consuming coffee and a variety of junk foods. I did some lab tests and told her to come back in three weeks when I had the results. In the meantime, I told her that if she changed her diet, she was likely to eliminate most of her problems. She dropped junk food, started eating salads and whole grains and taking multiple vitamins. I didn't want to prescribe any medications until I had the lab results. It wasn't necessary. When she came back three weeks later, she was much improved."

BREATHING TROUBLES AWAY

Given the clear connection between stress and psychological disturbances, it is not surprising that many physicians spoke of procedures such as meditation, yoga, deep breathing, and various forms of body work as treatment modalities for stress. This comment, from a Chicago psychiatrist, was typical: "A lot of us have found that if you can get a person to do hatha yoga and meditation on a regular basis, a lot of his emotional distress smooths out. Anxiety and depression have a physiological component, and these practices do something to the central nervous system that modulates it. People see and feel differently. For some, it's all they need. For others, it reduces the general tension so they can get to the deeper issues in psychotherapy."

Some of the procedures mentioned have become fairly commonplace in stress-reduction circles, although they still struggle for acceptance among most physicians. However, we were also told about more unusual techniques, some of which combine more than one approach and sound fairly strange—as with the method that a Santa Monica psychiatrist learned at the Esalen Institute and incorporated into his practice:

"Holotropic breathing, which was developed by Stanislav Grof, involves a degree of hyperventilation with some accompanying body work. Usually it's done in a darkened room with the eyes closed, and selected music is played in the background. The technique is said to give access to unconscious conflicts. More often than not, subjects seem to emotionally discharge the trauma of birth and the prenatal process. People have also reported what they felt were past life experiences. That's the best description I can give because I can't explain these phenomena in the usual psychological terms. Something happens that appears to be helpful, though the experience can also be very painful—screaming, crying, shaking, vibrating, and violent movement. This is done in a protected environment so people can't hurt themselves or others. Sometimes we get tremendous releases, leading to experiences of a transcendent nature—of oneness, a deep sense of well-being, and boundless energy."

According to the physician, the process takes place in three stages as the patient is guided through the rhythmic breathing: "You begin by energizing the system. The music is driving and fast, usually ethnic so you won't recognize it. It is important to just feel the musical energy. The fast music is followed by classical music and then spiritual music—perhaps a requiem or mass—that will tend to open the heart. The music corresponds to the three stages of the process.

"Then there's the body work. As the breathing becomes more rapid, what typically happens is that tensions develop in those places where suppressed emotions are anatomically bound. Instead of relaxation, the procedure seeks to intensify the tension in order to have it reach an orgasmic peak. Building up the tension produces a natural discharge of the blocked energy and symptomatic relief. The addition of specific external pressure helps the process."

He says the actual breathing instructions are simple: "You breathe a little faster and a little more efficiently than usual. If you forget to breathe, or you get lost in it, the monitoring physician will remind you."

We asked when, and with whom, he uses the technique. "I don't use it routinely," he replied. "I use it with people who are looking for more than just simple relief. This technique is often effective in exploring deeper issues or dealing with specific emotional problems.

For example, early sexual abuse or strongly resistant conditioning. I would use it with people who have been in therapy for a long time, with me or somebody else, going over the same material and somehow not getting anywhere."

When asked about his most memorable encounter, he recalled an ex-policeman: "He had a very powerful experience that included a lot of screaming and carrying on. He later described this trance state where he had been a prehistoric bird flying around and diving into the water. Then he went into a different sequence, where he was gnawing on the skull of something and biting into the brain, and this triggered an actual memory of something that had happened to him while on duty. He had shot someone, who ended up in a hospital presumably brain-dead. The man had been in a coma for three weeks, and one day, just as my patient walked into his room to see him, the man sat up, opened his eyes, pointed his finger at him, and screamed. Then he went back into a coma. It completely unnerved my patient. In the breathing process, he saw himself as a brutal predator.

"He's much better now, a lot more relaxed, less rigid, and more at ease with himself and his body. His throat spasms cleared up and his food goes down properly. Symbolically, I think this represented stuff he couldn't swallow."

When we asked him to explain how and why the technique works, he told us: "When things happen to you in real life, you don't necessarily experience them consciously. You can block them out because they were so horrible you can't deal with them. But the body remembers. What the breathing does is to emotionally replay these traumatic memories and to help resolve them. In the case of the policeman, he could remember the facts but not the emotional content, just as some people may recall being in a dangerous situation but without the accompanying fear. The role of the therapist is to help the patient relive the experience and process the emotional content in order to bring about some form of catharsis. With these breathing exercises, most patients report some degree of calm detachment from their ordeal and a profound sense of rising above their material concerns."

THE USE OF PSYCHEDELIC DRUGS

To our surprise, three of the physicians we interviewed wanted to talk about the use of psychoactive drugs that are currently banned from clinical use and research. An internist with faculty appointments at two leading universities told us that he had given LSD to terminally ill patients: "It was legal then. The first time was with a woman who was dying from ovarian cancer. I had read about how LSD was used in research experiments to ease the pain and suffering of the dying. I used the drug with four other dying patients. One typical comment they all expressed was, 'I'm looking down at that awful body and I'm anxious to leave it.' "

He told us about one patient in some detail: "She had never had LSD and wanted to have the experience because she knew she was going to die very shortly. It was the most bizarre thing I've ever seen. I wanted so much for her to have a liberating experience. I don't know if she did. She was lying down with earphones on, listening to music, and mumbling what sounded like gibberish for eight hours straight without stopping.

"I thought, 'This is a failure. What nonsense. What are we doing here? She's supposed to be in some heightened state.' Well, after her outpouring, she became quite peaceful. There was a sort of radiance about her. Not that I can prove it, but it seemed to me that all the gibberish was her processing material from her life, getting it out of her system. It left her clear and quiet and radiant. Two or three days later she died."

How did he explain the woman's experience? "There are those who believe that psychedelics can acquaint them with the near-death experience by specifically altering states of consciousness. These are assumptions, but researchers found that when LSD was given to terminally ill people, not only did the drug decrease the amount of pain medication that they needed but it also gave them the sense that death is not to be feared."

One psychiatrist told us she has had patients use the drug MDMA, also known by the colloquial term Ecstasy: "I was working with it when it was still legal. I first heard about it from a patient who was dying of cancer and was told that it could result in a spiritual experience. By the time I was able to get it, it was too late."

Saddened that she could not honor the request, the doctor decided to try the drug herself. Her experience was such that she has continued to use it with a few trusted patients, despite the possible risk to her professional standing: "My experience was that of an expanded state, where I was very loving, very free and compassionate—like a literal physical opening of the heart. I was able to communicate without reservations about things that I might not have felt safe enough to say otherwise, and I later learned that the person who was listening was able to *receive* my truth. That's what makes it so useful."

She recalled one particularly moving case: "A woman in her late fifties who had recently lost her husband struggled hard to work through that loss. Then, lo and behold, she developed cancer. She withdrew emotionally and became bitter and depressed. She lived about three months after the diagnosis. In the final stages, I gave her MDMA weekly. She became more accepting of her condition and her energy was greatly increased, which allowed her to do more things. She died peacefully at home, surrounded by friends. Without the MDMA she would probably have gotten weaker and died in the hospital, as millions of people do, in an alien, sterile environment. The drug changed the way she perceived death. She said she felt at one with the universe, more comfortable, peaceful, and more accepting."

When we asked the doctor why she chose to discuss an illegal substance, she replied: "MDMA was used by therapists for about fifteen years, discreetly. Then it got out of the hands of therapists. The authorities were afraid it was going to be the sixties all over again. The government didn't exactly make it illegal, they made it a Schedule I drug, which means that you have to get special permission to even do research with it. But the requirements are so stringent that it's effectively banned. There were hearings in Washington, and the administrative court judge ruled that research with MDMA should be encouraged. But the DEA took the position that the judge's opinion was only a 'recommendation.' It is still on Schedule I."

Another psychiatrist hoped that the laws would one day be relaxed so that qualified persons could do research on what he called *psycholytic therapy*. "The term 'psycholytic' was introduced as an alternative to 'psychedelic.' It means 'mind-loosening,' and it refers to substances that are thought to loosen the mind's defenses and dissolve ego boundaries. They have the potential to accelerate our understanding of the psyche and its effects on our health. An enormous amount of information, experience, and memory is hidden from us. Wouldn't it be more useful to have access to every aspect of ourselves? Granted, if the retrieval process was not controlled, we would be flooded with material from the unconscious. But if it were possible to selectively access this vast storehouse, it would be of the greatest help in psychotherapy and in every dimension of life. How can we exist optimally if so much of ourselves is denied to our consciousness? It seems an absurd dilemma. Yet, that dilemma is the basis of psychoanalysis and all other self-knowing disciplines.

"There's a bias in psychoanalytic therapy against using 'intrusive' methods to reveal the unconscious process, as if it's natural to lie on a couch and free-associate. There's no substance to this argument beyond the risk of using a method that hasn't been adequately evaluated. I think the taboo is really due to the fact that many of the drugs suggested for this purpose may also have the curious property of giving pleasure. We are an anhedonic society. Recently, the FDA said it was looking for a substitute for marijuana for treating glaucoma— one that doesn't make you feel so good. It's an astonishing and revealing statement. It seems that we have no compulsion about using drugs that may make us feel *bad*."

He acknowledged the potential for abuse, but felt that under proper supervision it was no different than for prescription drugs. "We have the ability to develop psycholytic agents that are powerful and acceptable, but we haven't put the effort into this as we have for other medical research."

A caveat

With the recognition of biochemical effects on mental conditions, everyone must be aware that the pendulum can swing too far in that direction. Just as in the heyday of psychoanalysis when there was a tendency to fit every abnormal mental condition into the Freudian model, we might now find a similar tendency to overvalue drugs in the treatment of psychiatric disorders. The great majority of our psychological ills are effectively handled by the mind's innate capacity to understand and correct itself, although in some cases the help of a psychotherapist is necessary. Psychoactive drugs are indicated for specific conditions, and are potent substances requiring specialized knowledge and experience. Doctors and patients alike would do well to exercise caution and common sense in their use.

CHAPTER 4

THE USE OF HERBS, NOSTRUMS, AND FOLK REMEDIES

In most pre-scientific cultures, medicine grew from a combination of trial and error, superstition, and circumstance. A cure might have been attributed to supernatural intervention. A remedy proffered by a priest or shaman might have been considered divinely inspired and therefore reliable. In some cultures, the touch of a king or spiritual leader was believed to have healing powers. In cultures that existed side by side with animals, the attributes of beasts were sometimes linked with remedies. An ailing person might be told to eat the heart of a lion or drink the blood of a carnivore. In some societies, the so called doctrine of signatures often applied; the appearance of a plant was said to reveal its medicinal properties. Hence, hepatica was given its name and used in the treatment of liver disorders because its leaves were shaped like a liver. Because the shape of its flowers resembled a head, "skullcap" was used to treat headaches. Some treatments were clearly of symbolic use only. In medieval Europe, where the Catholic church dominated human affairs, a root was held to have curative properties because it was shaped like a cross. Other traditions linked herbs to the astrological attributes of planets.

In places like Greece, Egypt, China, and India, sophisticated observations of the effects of various remedies were made and the results were codified in writing. Procedures that worked were added to the pharmacopoeia of the culture. Most of this early work centered on the medicinal use of herbs and plants. "The Lord hath created medicines out of the earth," says Ecclesiasticus, a conviction shared by most early societies. Many an unsung hero may have died along the way, but, through trial and error and careful observation, remedies were added to the body of information that was passed on, in writing or orally, to subsequent generations.

Much of the pharmacy of jungle, forest, and field stood the test of time, and dozens of remedies found their way to modern society through cross-cultural contacts and immigration. Some are with us in unrecognizable form, as drugs produced by major pharmaceutical companies whose chemists are able to synthesize the effective ingredients of certain healing plants. For example, early explorers observed natives chewing the tough bark of the chinchona tree and drinking a bitter liquid brewed from the same bark. From that bark, chemists developed quinine, an antidote to malaria. Similar observations gave us digitalis—a powerful drug used to regulate heart action—from the foxglove plant, morphine from the poppy, and many other standard medicines of the twentieth century.

Many treatments have survived in their original form as well, either as folk remedies passed along from one generation to another, or as maintained by professional herbalists. In the United States and Europe, herbal medicine continued to evolve in a limited way despite the dominance of allopathic medicine. Remedies were acquired from early contact with Native American healers, for example, as well as from cross-cultural exchanges between Western herbalists and their counterparts in Asia and the Third World.

A small but significant number of doctors we interviewed (perhaps ten percent) said they respected herbal and folk remedies enough to possibly recommend one if they were reasonably certain of its safety. A few had actually studied herbal medicine formally, while most simply added such remedies to their repertoire as they came their way, either through a colleague or a patient with ties to the culture where they are used. One proponent believed that herbs in their natural state were preferable to a processed medicine that has extracted the active ingredient. "Rather than isolating a specific chemical that's refined into a drug," he said, "you have the substance with all its co-factors intact and none of the side effects often associated with synthetic medicines."

The feeling among many of our physicians was that nothing with potential efficacy should be dismissed merely because it derives from a simpler culture or empirical observations. "Even if a remedy has only limited usefulness," said one physician, "or is totally useless except for the placebo effect, if it does the patient some good and it does no harm, then I think it deserves our attention. You never know where the next aspirin will come from." The active ingredient in aspirin, it should be noted, is salicylic acid. It is found as salicin in the bark of the willow tree, which members of certain cultures would chew to relieve pain. In fact, one doctor recommended powdered willow bark as a safe anti-inflammatory.

The doctors who discussed herbs and folk remedies with us ranged from those who use them to treat serious illnesses to those who limit their use to everyday ailments. We begin with an example of the former, a Los Angeles general practitioner who treats AIDS patients with a combination of lifestyle changes, drugs, nutrition, and herbs.

TREATING AIDS WITH HERBS

"I was already known as 'The Vitamin Lady' because I was prescribing nutrient therapy to patients with various physical problems. Then the gay guys gathered around and said, 'You have to do something. There's nothing for AIDS.' Basically, my philosophy is that the AIDS virus doesn't just strike out of nowhere and suddenly cause this major, horrible disease. There has to be a pre-existing immune system deficit. So I started thinking, if we could just correct some of the co-factors we could destroy the ability of the virus to wreak such havoc on people. So I went around the country to visit holistic physicians, trying to see what they were using. I don't believe that AIDS is necessarily a fatal disease.

"Some of the herbs we use are borage oil, a form of evening primrose oil that improves the functioning of white blood cells; Chinese cucumber root, which is said to kill cells infected by the AIDS virus; echinacea and goldenseal, which is an antibiotic combination; Saint-John's-wort, which increases energy and protects T-cells; and aloe vera. Aloe vera juice has been used as a natural medicinal compound for thousands of years in various cultures. One of its active ingredients is carrisyn, a large complex sugar molecule that stimulates the production of extra T-cells in patients with HIV infection. Carrisyn also stimulates production of the white cell known as the macrophage, and it helps make macrophages more potent." She says that certain symptoms of AIDS, principally fevers, fatigue, and night sweats, decrease or clear up with the use of carrisyn. (Another doctor told us that other countries are studying the use of carrisyn with AIDS patients.)

While her program has not been subject to scientific testing, she says she has treated more than 600 AIDS patients, and claims that a high percentage of them have survived in relatively sound condition far longer than would normally be expected. "The two-year survival rate with AZT [an FDA-approved drug said to be effective if used in the early stages of AIDS] is only about fifty percent. Mine is ninety-eight percent. In about three out of four cases the T-cells are starting to increase."

EVERYDAY AILMENTS

ALOE VERA

Of all the herbs and plants advocated by our respondents, the most frequently mentioned was aloe vera, a succulent with thick fronds filled with a gelatinous substance, which contains its reputed healing ingredients. "It has remarkable analgesic qualities," said one doctor. "It's been known ever since the time of Hippocrates. I grow it in my backyard. If I get a burn or a bee sting or a fly bite, or anything like that, I quickly snap open a leaf and put it on. It takes the irritation and the pain away." The same doctor also told us that aloe vera in liquid form is good for sore throats (you gargle with it) as well as for diarrhea and upset stomachs. "I use it with anyone who's got colitis, digestive problems, or dyspepsia—feeling burpy, an acid stomach, or flatulence. It's safe to give them aloe vera along with whatever else has been prescribed. It's soothing. As a matter of fact, a patient came to me last week with lower abdominal distress. After examining him, I said, 'Well, here, I've got an unopened bottle of aloe vera. Take it.' I saw him four days later, and he said the pain was all gone. It's safe, so why should I get into prescription medication in a case like that? I've also used it as a treatment for impotency. The patients say it revitalizes them."

Another advocate of aloe vera practices family medicine in Santa Fe. He said he finds it useful in treating gastrointestinal problems, particularly gastritis, diverticulosis, and duodenal ulcers: "I have them take a tablespoonful every two to three hours, maybe two tablespoonfuls, depending on how bad they are. I get some effective responses without the side effects of drugs or the dangers of using antacids, which have a lot of aluminum in them. Aloe vera juice or gel are very safe and have no adverse effects."

THE CASTOR PLANT

That same aloe vera advocate waxed even more enthusiastic about castor oil: "In India, the castor plant is thought to be a gift from God. It grows everywhere. They use it for a vast variety of illnesses, and they have pharmacopoeia shops devoted to castor plants. You buy the roots, stems, flowers, seeds, or leaves.

"I use castor oil for allergy treatment, rhinitis, bronchitis, bronchial asthma, and eczema—all of these do very well with five drops of castor oil each morning. I've had people take it constantly for thirty to sixty days and then take it a few times a week, depending on how bad their allergies are. I tell them to take it in juice or water. The easiest way is to take five drops on your tongue and wash it down with water. It doesn't taste bad and it really has a very positive effect."

He said he also uses the castor plant on external injuries: "I use castor oil packs for sprains, tennis elbow, and bursitis. You make the pack with a little flannel or cotton, soaked with castor oil. You wrap it around the inflamed joint, cover it with a piece of plastic to avoid staining anything, then you put a towel over it to keep it in place overnight. I cure more tennis elbows with that than I do with cortisone injections, without any adverse effects. I also use it on herpes zoster—I have the patient keep a castor oil pack on all the time. It immediately stops the majority of the burning and the pain, and it dries up the blisters."

A family physician in Arizona told us about castor oil poultices, a technique he said he learned from followers of Edgar Cayce, the reputed psychic healer: "It's great for liver detoxification. It can be used for vague abdominal or functional bowel problems. You take a piece of wool flannel and soak it in castor oil. You want to get a really good grade wool flannel and pure castor oil extract. You put the wool flannel in a pan and soak it in the castor oil and place it in the oven at a very low temperature for an hour to saturate the flannel. It'll be moist for months after that. You just put it on your abdomen and put a towel over it, and just lie in bed for an hour. It's very soothing. The theory is, the castor oil has some effect on what's called the visceral cutaneous reflex by penetrating and stimulating skin receptors that affect the organ below. The main thing is to do it over the area where the liver is. It seems to have a good effect on the liver."

CALMING CHAMOMILE

A number of doctors recommended chamomile tea for anxiety, insomnia, and other conditions where a calming influence is desired. A rural California physician had another use for the herb: "Chamomile tea can be used for viral conjunctivitis. You take a tea bag and soak it and keep it on the eye. People tend to get better. The person who taught me this was a guy in family practice. He had read it in a folk remedy book and tried it with a patient, and it worked. I thought it was kind of crazy and didn't pay attention to it until a couple of years later when a patient told me she had used it off and on over the years. I normally prescribe an antibiotic for conjunctivitis, but I've mentioned chamomile to certain patients who want to avoid drugs, for whatever reasons. I can say it's worth giving chamomile tea a try."

As for how to apply the remedy, he says you can purchase bulk chamomile tea at a health food store, brew it, and soak a handkerchief in it. "It has to be warm," he adds. "You rinse out the hanky, close the eye, lean back, and put it over the eye for five to ten minutes, two or three times a day. Maybe just putting warm cotton over the eye would work just as well, but there's something about using this herb that seems to help."

Some of the other uses of chamomile mentioned by doctors were for patients with calluses to soak their feet in chamomile tea, and for those with infections to drink it as an adjunct to other, more specific treatments. Also a poultice made of boiled chamomile flowers was said by one physician to relieve everything from aching muscles to sore throats. For nausea, another doctor recommended a tea made from mixing chamomile and peppermint.

HERBAL REMEDIES FOR THAT TIME OF THE MONTH

Herbal treatments for premenstrual syndrome were mentioned by a few physicians. "Women do not have to have PMS," one psychiatrist claimed. "There are all kinds of herbal remedies that can be easily procured at health food stores. I've had husbands and boyfriends ask me to treat women who have horrendous PMS. I change their diet a little, put them on some vitamins and herbs, and, in a few months, they are noticeably better, as long as they stick to the program. It's amazing that women still put up with it. The medical community does very little because it's a 'women's disease.' It's a sad comment on the medical establishment and our culture in general."

Another physician recommended a combination of herbs that he said has helped his PMS patients: "Their cramps are less severe, and sometimes they go away entirely. Their periods are more regular, and the patients are less subject to extreme moods. The ingredients that I find most effective are cohosh, capsicum, cascara sagrada, chamomile, damiana, dong qui, ginger root, and red raspberry, but the exact mixture depends upon the patient's problem."

FENUGREEK

A family physician who practices in the San Fernando Valley outside Los Angeles told us she swears by fenugreek seeds to treat sinusitis, bronchitis, and coughs: "The use of fenugreek goes back to the ancient Egyptians. I have the patients use one heaping tablespoonful of seeds to a quart of water. You boil this for ten minutes and then drink it, adding honey as a sweetener if you like. For bronchitis, I have them drink it four times a day.

"I first learned about this from someone I was dating. I had had surgery and afterwards I was getting sick a lot, colds, runny nose, always coughing, and a lot of congestion. It worked. I prefer fenugreek to over-the-counter cough medicines and expectorants. Those are not very useful. Codeine works by shutting off the cough reflex, and that's terrible. The body coughs in order to get rid of the irritant. You should take codeine only with a severe spasmodic cough or if you're coughing up blood. Fenugreek immediately releases the mucus, although it takes a while before you cough it all up."

A POTPOURRI OF PLANTS AND HERBS

One Los Angeles doctor was so effusive on the subject of plant-derived treatments that he poured forth a virtual catalog. Here is part of his interview:

"I've always been fascinated with plant-based medicine, so I picked up a bunch of remedies over the years. I use goldenseal and myrrh for a mouthwash, for example. When people get canker sores or a low-grade early gum infection, you make up a tea with two cups of water, a teaspoonful of goldenseal, and one of myrrh. You use it as a mouthwash two or three times a day, and in forty-eight hours your gums feel wonderful.

"A classic remedy for a cold is hot lemon water and cayenne. You take half a lemon and a quarter teaspoonful of red cayenne in a cup of hot water. You can put in a dollop of maple syrup to sweeten it. Mix it up, and drink it right down. Within half an hour you're sweating, but you wake up the next morning and you don't feel the cold anymore. There are other herbs for cold symptoms too, like licorice root, which is good for irritated throats, and garlic, which may be germicidal. Goldenseal is a classic. It really strengthens the nasal membranes. And echinacea is a great immune-system enhancer.

"I like using slippery elm powder for intestinal problems, like diarrhea, cramps, and gastritis. It's a white powder. You put a teaspoonful and a cup of warm water in a blender, and it turns up looking like hot chocolate. It coats the stomach lining and soothes the intestines, and it really helps. I'd reach for slippery elm before I would reach for an over the counter drug.

"Ginger is a really versatile herb. I use it in the early stages of a fever to help mobilize the body's defenses, and for heartburn and nausea, too. You can make a great ginger tea by scraping the root into hot water, or you can get powdered ginger in capsule form.

"Then there's fennel. I just had a patient with severe abdominal complaints—gas, bloating, belching. He went to a gastroenterologist who scheduled an expensive special procedure where a tube would be inserted into the intestines to see if there were tumors. In the interim I gave him some fennel tea, and in three or four days his symptoms were completely gone.

"When I get a patient who's anxious or nervous, there's a number of herbs I use to calm him down: passion flower, sand verbena, hops, lime blossom, chamomile, and especially valerian. Valerian is great for insomniacs.

"And if you ever get hemorrhoids, try using stoneroot. You can get it in capsules at health food stores, either under the name stoneroot or as collinsonia canadensis. It's said to strengthen the veins. You can also dab the hemorrhoid with witch hazel, preferably cold. Witch hazel has astringent qualities that cause blood vessels to shrink, and hemorrhoids are just swollen veins."

THE ESSENCE OF FLOWERS

No doubt the most unusual interview about plant-based remedies was with a Los Angeles family physician who uses, with selected patients, an esoteric system based on flower essences:

"They're especially effective for helping people with emotional problems. So many people come in with physical complaints, but much of this is due to stress and dissatisfaction with their lives. Flower essences seem to have a salutary effect on the emotions and the nervous system.

"Flower essences are specially prepared remedies. They take a fresh petal and allow it to sit in distilled water in the sun. The solar energy concentrates the essence of the flower into the water, and this is preserved with brandy. The remedies are taken as drops, under the tongue. They've been studied extensively, although not with case-control, double-blind experiments. There are standard remedies for particular emotional problems. Certain people are more responsive than others. I think it's partly a matter of belief and acceptance. The placebo effect is very powerful. But I think there is an underlying effect that is *not* placebo.

"One patient, for example, was very frightened, she was chronically fatigued, and unable to work. I gave her the remedy called 'fear energy release.' I had taken it myself once and had a very cathartic experience.

She took some here in the office, and she felt so much better she wanted more. Another woman had not been to a doctor in ten years and was terrified just to be in my office. She had severe anxiety because of an abusive relationship with her husband and a lot of family problems. I prescribed flower essences. She wasn't quite sure about it, but she called a few weeks later to thank me. She said she was incredibly changed, that people noticed it in her voice and her entire demeanor. She was calmer, happier, and more open to companionship."

The doctor told us the history of these flower remedies: "Rudolph Steiner, the mystic theosophist in the early part of the century, said that flowers were the astral body of a plant, and the astral plane is where the emotions are. The person who discovered the remedies was a British physician, Edward Bach. He would walk in woods and drink the dew from flowers that had been in the sun. He discovered that each flower evoked a particular emotion. Then he systematically gave the various essences to patients and noted their responses."

We asked how she thinks the remedies work. Her answer was rather metaphysical: "Physiologically, I can't explain it. Theoretically, they work on energy frequencies. When you put the flower in the water in sunlight, the energy of the plant goes into the water, which is a great medium for absorbing energy. An imprint of the flower's energy remains in the water, and the sun intensifies the reaction. So, when you take the drops, it's like a transfer of energy. The energy from the flower, now contained in the dilution, enters your body and has some kind of impact at a subtle level."

Whether or not there is any substance to her explanation would depend upon some as-yet-unknown scientific principle or at least my idiosyncratic rule, as described in the Prologue.

THE FOLKS WHO USE FOLK REMEDIES

A number of the doctors we interviewed were eager to talk about unusual folk remedies they've come across, either to share a little-known but efficacious nostrum or for the sheer delight of telling an interesting story. What follows are the best of that group.

A veteran internist, who teaches residents at a major medical school, told us of a remedy for arthritis that he heard about from his patients: "People come in and say, 'I've used paraffin dips. This old doctor told me about it years ago.' You melt paraffin in a can and dip your hands in the warm paraffin. As you pull your hands out of it, it gels and you have a glove of paraffin. You leave it on for a certain amount of time, wrapped in gauze. When you pull it off, it feels soothing—as long as you don't burn your hand on the paraffin."

A family practitioner working in the Midwestern countryside told us of a remedy used by veterinarians on cows, but which some of his patients use on themselves: "The most interesting thing I hear about here is Bag Balm. It's an antiseptic ointment used on the udders of a cow for inflammation and to prevent chafing and chapping, probably from overzealous milking. It's a real old-timer's remedy. I find a lot of patients who use it for various skin problems—abrasions, sunburn, itching, chapped hands or lips, that sort of thing. I've had people swear it's the best thing for their kids' diaper rash. It took a while before I saw the stuff, but somebody brought in a can of it. It feels a bit like Vaseline. It contains an antibiotic that's good for fungal and bacterial infections, and it has some lanolin, which is an oily substance derived from wool. I can't prescribe it because, strictly speaking, it's intended for use on animals and the FDA hasn't approved it for use on humans. But it seems to work, so I don't discourage patients from using it."

Here is an instance in which a doctor learned about a folk remedy under very fortuitous circumstances: "A woman had a tachycardia in my office. That's where the heart suddenly begins to beat very rapidly, as much as two hundred beats per minute. It starts suddenly and ends abruptly, although it can go on for hours. It's very frightening. I tried the usual things after I had her lie down: the Valsava maneuver, pressure, and inducing vomiting by putting a finger down her throat. I also tried carotid sinus massage. The only alternative left was drugs, but she was allergic to so many things I was hesitant to administer anything in the office. By this time, she was getting chest pains from her heart beating so fast. Then a Mexican-American woman, about twenty-four years old, who worked in the office told me that when her mother got this they'd put an ice cube in her mouth. Well, I knew that the vagus nerve has branches in the mouth and that it's connected to the heart, so I thought maybe there's something to this. I got an ice cube and put it in the patient's mouth, and, as soon as I did, the palpitations stopped. I had her hooked up to an EKG, so I know this really happened. And I told her, from now on, if you feel the palpitations, before you call me and before we put you on medication, take an ice cube and see what happens. It worked every time."

A Los Angeles general practitioner with twenty-seven years of experience came upon a folk remedy that she wishes she'd heard of sooner. It was for colic, the episodes of crying and irritability that afflict so many infants and drive their parents to distraction. "Doctors don't have very effective ways of stopping babies from crying all night," she told us, "but I had patients who would give the babies warm tea—usually made from manzanita or yerba buena—and they said it calmed the child down enough so the mother could go to sleep. I never observed any problems from this—they don't get diarrhea or any other reactions—so it's evidently a workable remedy. I've told several mothers about it, and most of them say it works."

A general practitioner, who had been practicing in Los Angeles for nearly thirty years at the time of our interview, said he has numbered among his patients members of immigrant groups who taught him native remedies: "I have patients who were from South America and the Middle East and other places, and the home remedies they used that I think have a modicum of veracity I'll go along with. For example, I had some Armenian patients who had kidney stones. They take the silk from an ear of corn and soak it in water and make a tea out of it, and then drink it. I did some chemical research on corn silk and found that it's high in phosphoric acids and rich in phosphates, which help dissolve kidney stones. I've seen with my own eyes X-rays of kidney stones having dissolved. For these patients, it's better than giving them phosphoric acid or phosphate tablets or elixirs. There is the emotional factor—a home remedy from their culture—and I reinforce it because I'm a fancy doctor and I've given it approbation by telling them, 'Yes, I understand why it works.' "

One of the more remarkable stories we heard was told by a doctor who has been practicing family medicine in Southern California since the 1960s. One of his patients, a young girl, had an ugly keloid formation on her chest: "A keloid is a smooth overgrowth of fibroblastic tissue that forms either in an area of injury or spontaneously. Certain people are predisposed to this condition. Whereas normal skin might produce a small scar, theirs will produce a huge, unsightly proliferation of scar tissue. In her case, the scar was so big it might have affected her psychologically the rest of her life. Well, she and her family are Puba Indians and they obtained a remedy from another Indian in their area, a tattoo artist, who gives it to her clients to help heal the scar tissue caused by tattooing. It's a powder, some formula I was not familiar with. They applied it to the scar, and it was the most fantastic thing I've ever seen in medical practice. The scar was reduced."

The doctor has since sent other scarred patients to the tattoo artist for the formula. He said he had no trepidation about providing patients with such an unusual referral. "See, you're not going to get involved in any liability. You can't make the scar any bigger. You can only make it smaller, and if this folk medicine does that, the patient's life will be changed for the better."

A clinical professor at a medical school in Southern California told us of a remedy he learned from his parents, who hailed from Turkey: "My dad used to make an onion poultice when I came home with a bruise on my leg. When there's a hard black and blue mark, you crush an onion—you beat it with a mallet—and put it in a towel or a piece of cloth, and apply it directly to the bruise. You leave it on overnight. There's an amazing reduction of the hardness, the pain, the swelling, the discoloration. I've used it on myself a couple of times when I've gotten a real bad bruise on the shin. And I've prescribed it to patients as well. Of course, you have to be selective about which patients you suggest it to. Some of them love this sort of thing, and they'd much rather do it than take a medicine or hear that there's nothing you can do.

"At first, I assumed that there was nothing unique about using an onion. I thought maybe applying a cool poultice with *anything* in it would work just as well. But it turns out that onions contain hyaluronidase, an enzyme that promotes a freer exchange of fluids between coagulated blood and surrounding cells, and a black and blue mark is caused by coagulated blood."

One doctor told us of several remedies that can be applied to the skin for bruises and other conditions: "I picked up one from a Hispanic patient. She had a really severe bruise on her arm. It was bleeding, and I applied the usual treatment. She came back a couple of days later, and it was almost healed. But she said it wasn't because of my medicine. She said she'd put a piece of papaya on it. So I tried it, and it worked quite well. I've also used different things for insect stings, like charcoal and vinegar. They seem to work. And honey. Honey is really good with burns. You can also use tea bags for canker sores and sunburn. Evidently, tannin, which is found in black tea, has pain-relieving properties. A bag of Lipton is great for a sty. Before you go to bed, you dip the tea bag in hot water and wring it out so it's not too strong. Then you lay the tea bag on the eye and put a towel over it to keep the heat in. When it cools, you dip it in hot water again, and repeat this a few times. The sty is usually gone by morning. The heat and the moisture plus the tannic acid act to open and drain the abscess."

Lemons were mentioned a couple of times. Drinking it with hot water and honey was recommended for sore throats and laryngitis, predictably, but it was also recommended for other uses. Here is an example: "I recommend lemon juice for people with congested sinuses, catarrhal conditions, or bronchitis. I have them take one drop of fresh lemon in each nostril and sniff it in. You can use an eye-dropper or snort the lemon juice out of your palm. Or, you can boil lemon juice and water and inhale the steam, and later drink the tea when it's cool enough. You do that two or three times a day, until your condition changes. If I have the slightest sign of a cold, I do that every hour until I've forgotten the idea."

And, of course, no chapter on folk remedies would be complete without a mention of the venerable chicken soup: "It was my grandmother's standby for the common cold and everything else that ails you," said a New York internist. "And now I find out that 'Jewish penicillin' might have some physiologic rationale behind it. Apparently, there was a study done in Miami Beach—where else, right?—and they found that chicken soup actually increases the flow of nasal mucus, which would definitely aid in the elimination of germs. Who knew?"

Finally, we received this fascinating response from a practitioner in Southern California, ninety percent of whose patients are Latino: "Generally speaking, I get two kinds of people: Westernized Latinos, who were raised and educated here, and recent immigrants. The longer the person has been here, the more comfortable he is with our forms of therapy; whereas, with the recent immigrants there tends to be a mixture of modern medicine and folk medicine. When you're working in a community like this, you realize that you can't dismiss their folk remedies. A lot of it is practiced in the back streets by the *curanderos,* the healers, who give people all kinds of things—herbs, chicken gizzards, poultices, witchcraft, various boiled things. Or they go to the herbal shop. They have all sorts of herbs for different conditions—they grind up this and that, and maybe some of them have active ingredients that we don't know about . . .

"I've seen them boil a tea, for instance, for a swollen foot, and put the poultice on it, and you don't know what it is because most of the time they have crazy names for these remedies. They put things in every orifice—their ears, their rectum, their vagina. Yet we have people who use these poultices and they feel absolutely marvelous. I'm not against it personally because most of the time there is no harm done if they feel better."

The physician added a note of concern that was repeated by many of our respondents: "I'm all for anything that works, but it's important to bear in mind that even a seemingly harmless folk remedy can do genuine harm if it keeps a patient from seeking a more efficacious treatment. I see that a lot in my area. A big part of it is economics. Many of the people here don't have insurance and can't afford to come to someone like me, so they use the remedies they can afford, unless it's something very serious. It's also family. The grandmother or the aunt says she knows how to cure something, and they go along with her. We used to get a lot of children with vitamin deficiencies because the older women would give them too many laxatives. They had a belief that if a child didn't have a bowel movement every day, something terrible would happen, so they'd give him mineral oil or olive oil as an enema, which would deplete the A and B vitamins."

That doctor's caveat is worth repeating as we close this chapter: a folk remedy, or any unusual treatment, for that matter, might be worth trying when no harm can result if it doesn't work. In the case of serious illness, however, they should not be used at the expense of other, more proven approaches. At the same time, they should not necessarily be dismissed as superstitions or the quaint remnants of backward cultures. Something that starts out as a seemingly naive or primitive remedy might one day be proven efficacious in a laboratory and packaged by a pharmaceutical company. With that in mind, we can only hope that humanity comes to its senses and stops the further wholesale destruction of native plant life, which has served for millennia as nature's apothecary.

CHAPTER 5

Your Foods Shall
Be Your Cures

"Your foods shall be your remedies, and your remedies shall be your foods." So stated Hippocrates, the Greek physician who has been revered through the centuries as the father of medicine. In the eyes of many physicians, the medical profession, whose oath is attributed to Hippocrates, has been remiss in heeding his injunction regarding the medicinal value of food. Until recently, few medical schools devoted more than cursory attention to the subject of nutrition. This has been criticized as everything from a careless or arbitrary omission to a politically motivated conspiracy. In my estimation, the historic neglect had more to do with the fact that diet is stubbornly resistant to scientific investigation. What we call the metabolic mill—the course food takes from ingestion through digestion to elimination—is so complex, our diets are so mixed, and the components of individual foods are so multifarious that determining the potential of any diet to cause or cure disease is an extremely complicated task. In addition, the tremendous variation among individuals and cultures in their biological response to foods makes it exceedingly difficult to make universal cause-and-effect statements.

For these reasons, the field of nutrition has always been beset by conflicting theories and claims, and never more so than in recent years when speculation has reached new heights. As any reader of health publications knows, there are as many diets claiming to represent the truth as there are religious sects. In the past decade, a storm of activity has centered around nutrition, with medical schools and research labs taking the subject much more seriously than they have ever done. Out of all this has emerged enough scientific evidence to clearly establish the role of diet as a contributing factor in heart disease, diabetes, colon cancer, vitamin deficiencies, and other conditions, and for recommended dietary regimens to have been dramatically altered in the direction of less fat and sugar and more fiber, fresh fruits, grains, and vegetables. Perhaps predictably, these developments are precisely what radicals were advocating in the last three or four decades.

While medicine has never been more nutritionally oriented, a large number of physicians still feel that the mainstream has not gone nearly far enough, either in its recommendations or its acceptance of the role of nutrition in causing or curing diseases. The excerpts that follow represent the opinions of doctors who would go *much* further in attributing both toxic and healing properties to food, and who, in their practices, commonly treat patients with various nutritional procedures.

We begin with three physicians who made major changes in their career orientations as a result of experiences involving nutrition. The first is a retired pediatrician in the Northwest who, in the 1960s, discovered a connection between food sensitivities and various symptoms: "I began to realize as time went by that much of the stuff that we got in medical school was in some way influenced by the pharmaceutical industry. We were supposed to become good diagnosticians, and then the pharmaceutical company would supply the drug. I said, 'Gee, that's a nice neat setup. We just make the diagnosis and then write up the prescription. Never a thought as to why the kid got sick in the first place.' So, when I discovered that my own kid wet the bed because he drank milk, and kids with ear trouble would get better when I took them off milk, I began to wonder about all the rest of the stuff we learned in school. Do I have to redo all that training? Well, obviously not. But at least, it opened up the door for me. I found a whole other world out there. I began to talk to alternative health practitioners and found they had good results, sometimes even better than what medical doctors were getting. We had been kind of hood-winked in school. We were told that anybody who wasn't an M.D. was a quack." He went on to a career that mixed traditional pediatrics with a variety of offbeat procedures, some of which we will hear about later.

Our next convert is a young cardiologist whose transformation occurred around 1980: "I was frustrated because I realized that no one was getting healed of cardiovascular disease. There were no cures, only treatments for the symptoms. Bypass is not like an appendectomy. If you don't reverse the risk factors, if your cholesterol level stays high and you're stressed and not exercising, the grafts will also get athero-sclerosis. The turning point was when I saw what Nathan Pritikin was doing with cardiovascular patients, using just diet and exercise. Ninety percent of the hypertensives that came in went off their medication. I'd never seen that. I was under the impression you had to use anti-hypertensives to lower blood pressure, and right before my eyes the blood pressure went down and they *had* to get off the medication, or it would be too low."

The doctor ended up establishing a private cardiology practice that features dietary recommendations calling for much less fat than the usual thirty percent of caloric intake, as well as lifestyle modification and psychotherapy. Our next story is from a general practitioner who made even more radical changes in his personal eating habits and his practice. They began with what he terms a dramatic epiphany:

"I was a resident on the cardiovascular and anesthesia service, which deals with the heart and blood vessels. I was making my rounds one night for the next morning's surgery. One patient was a very nice man, but grossly obese, who was scheduled for a coronary bypass. I took a blood sample and left it at the nurses' station while I finished my rounds. When I got back to take the blood down to the lab, well,

I couldn't believe my eyes. Normally, when you draw blood and let it sit for an hour, it separates into two parts: the clot settles to the bottom and the serum rises to the top. And normally serum is transparent yellow—you can see right through it. This blood looked like Elmer's glue. It was thick and greasy white. It stuck to the sides of the tube when I shook it.

"I asked the patient if he had eaten before he came to the hospital. He said he had had a cheeseburger and a milk shake. I realized that what I was looking at in the blood tube was all that fat from his meal. It's a well-known phenomenon called lypemia—it means fat in the blood. After a meal it stays in your blood for about four hours before your liver can clear it out, and that surge of fat after a meal is when the arteries start clogging up. I had read about this in pathology, but it was the first time I had seen it so graphically.

"The next morning I took him to the operating room and put him to sleep, and the surgeon opened up his chest and started reaming out these big long yellow sausages of fatty material from the man's arteries. Well, I was watching all that and remembering what his blood looked like the night before, and I made the connection. That's what this stuff is. That's the fat from all the animals this man has eaten. It may be out of sight and out of mind, but it's not out of the arteries. That was a very profound lesson for me.

"When you send this yellow material to a pathologist for a chemical analysis, the report always comes back: saturated fat and cholesterol. It never comes back: remnants of broccoli, rice, and tofu. That made a big impression on me because I was drinking a quart and a half of grade A milk a day, I was eating cheese by the chunk, and I had a spare tire of twenty pounds of fat around my waist.

"The experience made me wonder if eating animal products is necessary at all. So I read books on nutrition, physiology, and biochemistry, and when I was satisfied that I wouldn't be nutritionally deficient if I eliminated animal products for a while, I cleaned out my refrigerator, bought some cook books, and started experimenting."

Meanwhile, he told us, two other significant events occurred in the hospital. "First, the patient was discharged after a rough postoperative course. When he left, all he had was an appointment to see the surgeon to get his stitches out. Nobody told him anything about his diet—not the nurse, not the dietician, not the surgeon. Nobody talked about all that yellow stuff in his arteries, and what was going to happen to the nice new grafts we put in if he kept eating a lot of fat. Within three to five years, those grafts will be clogged and he'll be back on the operating table, or dead. Also, what about his other arteries? It's a total body disease. They weren't getting at the core of the problem.

"Then came the clincher. I had just finished with a bypass case and was going through the cafeteria line behind the surgeon. He was a big, fat man, and I watched him load up his tray with hamburgers, french fries, and cheesecake. I thought, I'm in a Fellini movie. This is bizarre. What does this man think he's been doing for the past five hours? What does he think all that yellow gook was he took out of that man's arteries? It's an old biblical adage: 'It shall happen to thee and to thee, but not to me.' I thought, I'm working in the wrong building. I'm in anesthesia. I put people to sleep all day. I want to help people wake up. I went to the head of my department and said, 'I'm going back to general practice and see if I can't keep people off these operating tables.' "

He ended up in a small practice in Florida, where he installed a kitchen in his office and brought in a vegetarian cook to teach patients how to eat well without animal products. "A good ninety percent of what walks through the G.P.'s office door is related to diet," he believes. "Obesity, high blood pressure, clogged arteries, sore joints, cancers, allergies—the majority of those come from running too much fat, salt, and animal protein through your bloodstream. I get corroboration of that in the following way. I tell people to do two things: eat like I show you and take a walk every day. Come back in a week, get on the scale, take your blood pressure. People who do it notice something wonderful. Week to week there is a downward progression of numbers on their chart. Their weight goes down. If they had high blood pressure, it comes down. If they had high cholesterol, it drops six to eight points a week, and if they had gout, the uric acid level goes down.

"Usually I end up lowering the dosage of medication for hypertension, diabetes, or arthritis. When their weight starts coming down, they complain, 'I'm getting dizzy when I stand up,' and I check their pressure and see that they don't need as much medication. Same with my adult-onset diabetics. As they get leaner, they have more insulin circulating in their blood to do what it should be doing. They start complaining of headaches and dizziness, and sure enough, they have *low* blood sugar, and I have to reduce their anti-sugar medication. I was told that diabetes never goes away, but it does. I was told that high blood pressure never goes away, that you have to take pills the rest of your life. Nonsense.

"I've also had a lot of success with inflammatory conditions. People would say, 'My joints don't hurt anymore. My nose stopped running. I haven't had to use my asthma medication in two weeks. My psoriasis cleared up.' I had no idea why those things should happen, but I suspect that when people eat animal protein, small fragments get into their bloodstream fairly intact. The immune system responds, and suddenly they have antibodies cruising their bloodstreams looking for animal protein that is found in their skin, joints and nasal and bronchial membranes. That sets off inflammatory reactions. We call these rheumatoid arthritis, excema, asthma, etcetera. When I get patients off animal protein, a lot of these inflammatory reactions begin to subside. Not every case, of course, but a lot of them."

We pointed out that many people contend that animal protein contains nutrients we can't get from other sources. "That's a nutritional old wives' tale," he replied. "The fact is, all eight amino acids we require to build our structural proteins are found in more than sufficient amounts in plant protein. Corn, rice, and wheat are complete proteins. There are two key differences that tilt the balance in favor of vegetable protein. One, animal muscle has a large amount of sulfur-containing amino acids. As these amino acids are metabolized, the blood becomes more acidic and causes calcium to dissolve. So, one problem with eating animal protein is that you start eliminating your calcium when you urinate, and this is a chief culprit in osteoporosis. Plant protein is more alkaline. Two, plant proteins are absorbed slowly, while meat protein is absorbed very quickly. There's a sudden flood of protein through the kidneys, which can clog up the kidney filters. That's why one of the chief causes of renal failure seems to be a high-meat diet."

We asked if he believes a vegetarian diet is right for everyone: "I strongly suspect that if I put a hundred people on a pure vegetarian diet and check them six months later, ninety will be doing wonderfully—they will be leaner, have lots of energy, their bowels will work better, etcetera—but ten will tell me they're not doing so great. They don't have much energy, are hungry all the time, and they're dreaming of steaks. If someone would endow me, I would start an institute of vegetarian studies to study these people. Something in their body has a need that is met by animal products. Maybe certain people's genes make it easier for them to metabolize animal protein. Also, when some people become vegetarians, they're careless about getting enough protein, so you have to add some beans or pasta. If they're motivated, you can usually find the right combinations for them."

SUPPLEMENTS AND DIET

A number of doctors advocated the use of vitamin and mineral supplements. Most were moderate in their view, suggesting a multivitamin as a kind of insurance against the failure to obtain needed nutrients in one's diet. Others were more radical, actually treating illness with massive doses of vitamins, or with minerals, amino acids, and other supplements. Among those with strong opinions about the value of supplements was a New York general practitioner: "The conventional wisdom is that all you have to do is eat 1200 calories a day of the four food groups and you will have all you need. It's based on the notion that the Recommended Daily Allowance has sufficient leeway, so, if you get that much, you're adequately nourished. To me, the error in thinking has been twofold. One, the RDA is defined as the amount necessary for healthy Americans, so you have to define what you mean by 'healthy Americans.' Two, are we talking about the amount necessary to prevent deficiency disease, or are we searching for a nutritional foundation that allows a reasonable approach to optimal health? I believe that optimal health is a better standard and a more desirable objective. It brings up the question, what does 'normal' mean? We can't look at averages as being normal."

He drew a parallel to what happened with other notions of normalcy. "It used to be that the normal scale for cholesterol was 150 to 300 because ninety-five percent of the population fell between that range. But who says that ninety-five percent of the population is normal in a healthy sense? And they weren't looking at the population as a whole; they were looking at that portion of the population that agreed to give blood, and most of those people were in doctors' offices because they were ill. But that's what it was until a few years ago. Suddenly, people said we have to stop kidding ourselves that a cholesterol count of 300 is all right. As a good friend of mine said, 'The average man with the average cholesterol has an average chance of having an average heart attack.' Now we teach people that their cholesterol should be below *two* hundred." He believes that future studies will force a similar modification of what we now consider adequate vitamin and mineral consumption.

VITAMIN C

When you think of vitamins, you usually think of Vitamin C for the common cold, a treatment that has been controversial ever since Linus Pauling first expounded it in the 1960s. One of our respondents was an early proponent of Vitamin C—and not just for colds. He recounted his history: "In 1968 I was a happy orthopedic surgeon, but I got frequent colds. If I went three months without a cold, I was lucky. I also had seasonal hay fever all my life. I heard Linus Pauling give a talk about Vitamin C and the common cold, and I was willing to try anything, so I took it in the form of powdered ascorbic acid—one teaspoonful four times a day. I didn't realize how much that was, but it turned out to be four grams four times a day. Astonishingly, my hay fever went away. About fifteen minutes after taking it, my nose would clear up. If I didn't take my next dose, it would get clogged up again.

"Now, I'm not saying it does that all the time for everybody, or that it's as easy for me now; I don't get perfect relief, but I don't have to take antihistamines much anymore. After nine months, I caught a cold, and I noted that fifteen minutes after taking ascorbic acid my symptoms went away and they stayed away for about an hour, and then they came back. So I took another dose. I was forty at the time, and I had what would now be called chronic fatigue syndrome. The ascorbic pepped me up. I started taking sixteen grams a day regularly. I found that cold symptoms also went away fifteen minutes after taking it. An hour later they would return, and I would take another dose and another dose, and so on. By the end of the day, I realized that I'd taken about fifty grams. Previously I discovered that when I exceeded this dose, it would cause diarrhea, but while I had my cold, it didn't. Then, as I recovered from the cold, the tolerance for ascorbic went back down to normal."

Curious about the shift in diarrhea symptoms, a common side effect of too much vitamin C, he attempted to reproduce his experience with select patients: "I found that when a person was sick, his bowel tolerance to the ascorbic acid went up. He could take more without getting diarrhea. The tolerance was in proportion to how sick he was. Over a few years I found that the average person can take ten to twenty grams in twenty-four hours before it produces diarrhea. With a mild cold, a person can take thirty to sixty grams, with a bad cold maybe a hundred grams, and with severe diseases, like mono or viral pneumonia, sometimes they can exceed two hundred grams without producing diarrhea. When the patient gets well, the tolerance goes back to normal. It seems to be a good idea to adjust the dosage according to bowel tolerance."

The doctor eventually became a major proponent of Vitamin C: "I believe that using massive doses of ascorbic acid will amount to a paradigm shift in medicine. We're talking about something that will change how all of medicine is practiced. Nobody uses enough. Pauling talked about two grams an hour. That will take out what I call a twenty-gram cold. To me, a bad cold is a fifty-gram cold, a severe cold is a hundred-gram cold. By that, I mean a cold that allows you to take a hundred grams in twenty-four hours the first couple of days before it produces diarrhea. Most people get minor colds, and they take two grams an hour, and it knocks it out, and they become convinced that Vitamin C cures the common cold. People don't go to doctors for twenty- or thirty-gram colds, they go for seventy-five- or a hundred-gram colds."

While most people have heard about the use of massive doses of Vitamin C for colds, few are aware that the substance is being used for other, far more serious, conditions. For example, we heard this story from an immunologist: "I had a patient in a hospital with severe burns on both legs that destroyed the skin and the muscle layers in big three-by-six-inch patches. I called in a plastic surgeon to see if he would graft them. He said, 'You're doing fine, keep her on the antibiotics, and we'll check her in a couple of weeks.' Well, after a couple of weeks it still didn't look like it was ready for grafting, so we kept her on the antibiotics. Another week went by, and the woman said, 'I've been here for three weeks. Can't you do anything?' I didn't want to rock the boat, but I did it anyway. I came in late one night and wrote on the chart, 'Ascorbic acid (Vitamin C), one thousand milligrams, four times a day, plus zinc sulfate, two hundred and twenty milligrams, three times a day.' The next morning I went into the hospital and the plastic surgeon was furious. Well, to make a long story short, in four to five days, the gap, which previously had not improved, closed up by fifty percent and she never needed any grafting. It just closed by itself."

To our surprise, three doctors we spoke to advocated the use of supplements, particularly Vitamin C, for viral disorders such as hepatitis, mononucleosis, and even AIDS: "When I heard about AIDS in 1983, I felt a social obligation," one doctor told us. "I gave intravenous ascorbate to some guys. It was amazing. You could see Kaposi's sarcoma begin to fade, and there was no question that it ameliorated the disease. We also gave them zinc, manganese, chromium, selenium, and B vitamins and Vitamin E, and we insisted that they quit eating sugar. I found we can delay the onset of the secondary complications and almost double their life expectancy. I'm counting only the ones who were really cooperative. I haven't kept formal statistics."

The Los Angeles physician who, in chapter four, spoke about treating AIDS patients with herbs also uses nutritional supplements, including the maximum dose of C that the patient can tolerate before getting diarrhea. "Nutrients can take the place of drugs if you take them in large enough quantities," she contends. "And for the most part, they don't have the same bad reactions. It's very hard to overdose on nutrients. For most people, the maximum dose of C is about eighteen grams. One orange has only thirty milligrams—you couldn't eat 600 oranges. You have to use concentrated supplements and/or do it intravenously."

In addition to Vitamin C, she uses Vitamin A, and a B vitamin formula she originated: "I make up the formula here from about thirty ingredients. It gets around the problem of absorption that AIDS patients have with B Vitamins. It has been my professional opinion, and I've been trying to convince other doctors about it for a long time, that some of the dementia, anemia, and some of the tingling sensations in the hands and the feet are not due to the AIDS virus or to AZT. They're due to B vitamin deficiencies that are not recognized by traditional doctors. I'm proud to say that not one of my patients this year has had any dementia, and that is very unusual for this population. Other doctors have said, 'Either you're lying or I want to know what you're doing.' "

A third doctor discussed the use of Vitamin C for AIDS, and his story was especially moving because his only patient was his son: "He tested HIV positive a few years ago, and then he got pneumocystis last year. It just about took his life. He was back in town by then, and my wife and I snuck down to the hospital and had this huge syringe full of Vitamin C. She stood at the door so nobody would come in, and I stuck him with it and put ten grams in each muscle. I think we saved his life. It kind of pulled him through. It helped his immune system just enough. I did it once a day for three or four days. They were treating him with an antibiotic, which helped, but it wasn't the complete cure. He still had this terrible, racking cough."

At the time of our interview, the doctor's son was out of the hospital and living at home, where he takes massive doses of vitamins: "He's 140 pounds. He's scrawny. He's got a Kaposi's lesion on his cheek now, so he knows he's going to die. But, we've kept on. He should have died a year and a half ago, but he gives me credit for his 'borrowed time' because I give him an intravenous Vitamin C every two weeks and a B-12 shot every day or two. My son knows that I'm a little radical, but he knows that what I've been doing has helped him."

IF IT SMELLS GOOD, DO IT

The pediatrician we met at the beginning of the chapter told us about a most unusual method of determining which supplements a patient needs. It sounds bizarre, but it's reminiscent of the observation by researchers that children who have not been influenced by family or television commercials will, if presented with a variety of foods, select those that their bodies need at that time. Said this doctor: "I got a call from a chemist who worked with animals for twenty-five years and who noticed that animals don't eat anything unless it smells good. That is probably why the nose is in front of the mouth. If it doesn't smell good, you say, 'Whoops, I'm not going to eat that.' So he figured it must be the same with humans, and he put together this program. It consists of twenty bottles, each with a different vitamin and mineral. You smell each one. If it smells good, you take it. If it smells bad, you don't. He correlates this with a blood test and files it in a computer. I've been doing it for three years, and it's just fascinating. For instance, my calcium level should be between 8.5 and 10.5. That's a really wide variation. So, I have my blood tested, and my calcium is about 8.8—low, but not wiped out. And when I go through the kit during that time, the calcium smells good to me. But if I've had some milk or cheese or something with calcium in it, the next day that calcium bottle smells like used kitty litter, so I don't eat it.

"The point is, we don't make a mistake because it's sort of immediate feedback and control. He pointed this out to me. If you had a meal of oysters, which have a lot of zinc, and then you were offered an apple or an apricot, you'd tend to choose the apricot because there's more manganese than zinc in an apricot. We tend to balance our dietary intake. For example, my wife loves the smell of ammonium chloride. She's very alkaline. I give her three of those tablets morning and evening, depending on the smell. If it doesn't smell good, I don't give her any."

Evidently, patients purchase the kits in order to test themselves so they know which supplements to take each day. The doctor told us some case histories: "There was a twenty-year-old woman who was depressed all the time for no apparent reason. I used to give her vitamin shots, and they worked for a while, but then they became ineffective. Well, time passed and I began using the smelling kit. She came back to see me when she was thirty and married. She still had these episodes of depression. So I had her go through the kit, and she smelled the B-1 and said, 'This smells like I have my head in the toilet.'

She didn't need B-1 except maybe one pill every three months. But, the rest of the B vitamins smelled good or neutral, so she takes them every day, and she does not get depressed."

He told us about a five-year-old child who has convulsions and was helped, oddly enough, by drinking vinegar: "He'd had the convulsions since he was two, and the doctor couldn't stop them without sedating the kid with drugs. So we got a blood test, and it was extremely alkaline. If he drank a pint of vinegar a day, he would have only two convulsions instead of twelve. He had to keep this up just to make sure he stayed in an acidic state instead of being so alkaline. His doctor told his mother, 'If you treat him with this crazy stuff, I won't be your doctor anymore.' So they stopped and tried to find some other drug. But the vinegar was working.

"Let me tell you how I help my wife get a good night's sleep. When she's asleep, I'll go in with this bottle of ammonium chloride. I'll wake her up and have her smell it. If she says, 'I don't smell anything,' I give her some, and she has this nice, nice sleep. If I forget to, or if I'm out of town, she'll wake up at two in the morning with terrible cramps in her foot and leg. The idea is that the ammonium chloride is a salt, it's an acidifier. It frees up the calcium so it's soluble and can get into the system. A lot of cramps are due to low calcium."

MULTIFARIOUS SUPPLEMENTS

Some advocates of nutritional supplements seem to have a veritable arsenal of vitamins, minerals, and amino acids that they draw from for a variety of ailments. One such is a California doctor with a history of bumping up against authorities: One of his chief interests is excessive blood clotting and the complications he says ensue from that condition: "We did a study with patients and found that seventy percent of those who had circulatory complaints had excess clotting, and there was a seventy percent correlation to abnormal cholesterol HDL ratios. We developed a blood test that detects excess clotting, and when I find it, I adjust the patients' diets and have them take fish oils because we found them to be most effective in breaking up the clotting. Some people can't tolerate it, so I try other things such as primrose oil and combinations of things like Vitamin B-6 with magnesium and Vitamin E.

"People come in with headaches. Nineteen out of twenty are due to excess clotting. You take some fish oil, and a half hour later the headache is gone. Sometimes the fish oil is not enough. Just the other day a lady came in. She had had terrible headaches for two or three weeks. We gave her sublingual heparin, which is a natural anti-clotting substance made from an animal source. Her headaches went away in five minutes. Heparin is great for chest pain, too. A lot of people with fatigue have excess clotting, too. I find that fatigue is the most common complaint. The clots block oxygen to the tissues, which makes the person tired and sometimes depressed. You give them heparin, the clots break up, and it's a little oxygen rush. There might be some endorphin release, I don't know. Sometimes they get euphoric. I put them on minerals too, primarily magnesium, zinc, and calcium. Zinc activates the thyroid and helps a sluggish liver. And they respond very well." It should be noted that heparin in general medical use demands careful supervision and continuous blood monitoring.

One family physician in Los Angeles was a veritable encyclopedia of food-oriented treatments. To complete this section, we culled the most interesting statements from his lengthy interview:

"I've had a lot of success treating herpes. In Chinese medicine they believe if you are too acidic, you can get oral herpes. I think it's also true of vaginal herpes. If your body is too acid, you're more vulnerable to the virus. I would say that ninety percent of it is due to overindulgence of acidic foods and juices. So my therapy is to eliminate everything that's acid for one week. That includes citrus fruit, pineapples, cherries, tomatoes, coffee, things like that. There is a marked improvement. Also, the Chinese use winter melon soup, which balances out the acids for some reason, and the herpes in the mouth will disappear.

For herpes simplex, the fever blisters or cold sores people get on their lips, one thing that works great is lysine. It's an amino acid that can be found in health food stores.

"To fight off infections, I give them seventy-five milligrams of zinc a day. If it's a bacterial infection, I have them eat a lot of yogurt. I tell arthritis patients to take a teaspoonful per day of cod liver oil; it seems to relieve the pain quite effectively. Calcium supplements and calcium-rich foods are really important for nerve-related conditions—high blood pressure, anxiety, insomnia. I think they're also good for patients with high cholesterol counts, as is niacin. It lowers cholesterol, and it also helps people with circulatory problems. I had a patient with inner ear problems who would get dizzy spells and tinnitus, and the ear specialists couldn't do a thing except rule out a tumor. The niacin helped her a lot. It increases the blood flow to the head. I also recommend niacin to diabetics, along with chromium supplements, to help them manage their blood sugar. I discovered a great treatment for dysmenorrhea [painful menstruation] when a patient with an extreme case came to me. She also happened to have very low blood sugar, especially during menstruation, so I began treating her with fruit juice a few days ahead of her period to help the blood sugar problem, and it turned out we could prevent her dysmenorrhea. I later heard that a lot of women with functional dysmenorrhea have low blood sugar when they start their periods."

HARMFUL FOODS

Naturally, foods can harm as well as heal. A large number of doctors mentioned this, condemning the usual suspects like fats, sugar, salt, and caffeine. Others talked about allergies, going considerably further than mainstream medicine in attributing disease conditions to food sensitivities. One such physician practices in a Los Angeles suburb: "I happen to believe that almost everybody is food-intolerant or allergic to some of the foods they're eating. We have an abundance of food here, and people are not very selective or careful. There are foods that can be great from a nutritional point of view yet make a particular person sick. For example, someone had nasal congestion, hemorrhoids, gas, and abdominal pain. I used a skin testing technique, and he turned out to be allergic to milk, wheat, and eggs, and that's what he ate for breakfast every morning. His mother gave him a healthful breakfast, but it had been making him sick all his life.

"I saw a teenage boy who had severe headaches. He'd been in a hospital and had had brain scans, X-rays, and lumbar punctures, and there wasn't any response. I put him on a special diet, and within a couple of days his headaches went away. He turned out to be milk-allergic. I had a young female patient who had six to eight episodes a year of what was considered cystitis, a urinary tract infection. She also had respiratory allergies and asthma, and I was giving her shots and medication, but I didn't think there was a connection between her allergies and her urinary system. Then I read an article about a case of recurrent bladder infections that were actually due to food allergies. Her mother agreed there was nothing to lose, so we put her on a special diet, her infections went away, and she didn't need cystoscopies every few months."

Another allergist became a convert to a controversial approach to testing and treatment. "It's called provocation neutralization," she said. "It's far more precise and more time-consuming, but it is also far more effective. Allergy is an unsuspected, unrecognized, underrated cause of illness in any part of the body. Many problems that are labeled idiopathic, meaning the cause is unknown, could very well be allergy-related."

In the early stages of her conversion to a new procedure, she set out to document its value: "I went to the dietitians at the hospital, and we worked out a two-week diet that eliminated highly allergenic foods. Then I went to a couple of pediatricians and got a group of twenty-four hyperactive patients who had been on Ritalin, and I put them on my two-week diet. About two-thirds of them stopped being hyper-active. They responded, in essence, to the diet." She explained that it eliminated foods she considered major allergens: milk, wheat, eggs, chocolate, and corn sugar, along with dyes and preservatives. "I added the foods back one at a time when the patients were better, and I found that one food would cause headaches, another would cause hyperactivity, another ear debility, another enuresis [bed wetting], and another caused nasal congestion. Different foods caused different symptoms in different children, but the symptom was consistent in the same patient. In testing the patient with these newer methods, I could produce the same symptoms, or similar symptoms, to the ones that were caused when the child ate the foods. Bed wetting is fre-quently milk or juices. Milk tends to cause nasal congestion, ear infections, bed wetting, and digestive problems like constipation, diar-rhea, and a bloated belly."

A family doctor in Northern California learned, from his patients, about a connection between certain substances and fibrocystic breast disease: "There are a lot of women with lumpy breasts that are often more tender around their period. I didn't realize there was a treatment for it. I thought it was just a natural condition of womanhood. But some patients told me that certain foods would make it worse. I thought they were crazy, but I have since found that they were absolutely correct. It's very humbling. The items they mentioned were coffee and chocolate. Now, both of them contain Xanthine com-pounds, and later I read in the medical literature of a connection between Xanthine and fibrocystic breasts. Xanthine compounds seem to exacerbate the cysts.

"I had never been able to treat it before. I would say, 'It's too bad you've got that.' And sometimes it can be a painful condition. Now I see major improvement when I advise patients to stay away from coffee and chocolate. Also, certain drugs have Xanthine. One of the classic asthma drugs is a Xanthine derivative. I'm more aware of that with female asthmatics. I'll tell them, 'Your breasts may become enlarged, but don't be alarmed. They'll return to their usual size once you're off the drug.' "

CLEANSING ELIMINATION

Traditionally, medical practitioners have viewed the gastrointestinal system not only as the means of supplying nutrients to the body but of *removing* what is unwanted. Hence, virtually every culture seems to have developed methods of cleansing and detoxification. Enemas, for example, have been in use at least since Hippocrates noted that certain birds used their beaks to squirt water into their rectums. We found in our interviews a number of provocative suggestions for cleansing the intestinal tract.

We begin with a Los Angeles practitioner who was unconventional long before anyone thought of terms such as alternative or holistic. His interest in the healing properties of foods and plants, he said, dates back to the Great Depression, when he was fed whole grains and helped his family grow organic vegetables: "It taught me where foods come from. My parents would take white bread and roll it into a ball and bounce it off the floor, saying, 'This is not food for humans.' My mentors were the original proponents of nutritional medicine, like Gaylord Hauser and Carleton Fredericks. I was using brewer's yeast, vitamins, liver tablets, etc. in the fifties. It wasn't even on the fringe then, since no one knew it was there."

He said he learned his first nutritional lessons from his mother: "The first was to eat the greatest variety of foods possible. The second was to make sure the colon is clean. She saved me a lot of night calls. When I first went into practice, people would call and say their babies had high temperatures, and I'd say, 'All right, this is what you're going to do: give him a cooling enema, and if the temperature is still up in a half hour, then you call me and I'll come.' I never made a house call for a baby that I can remember. Instead of giving them aspirin and this and that, that's the advice I gave them because if the temperature didn't come down, there was still time to do something about it. When a child is sick, everything is off, and in a baby the intestinal track is very, very important.

"I don't often prescribe enemas for adults. I tell people to clean out their colons, but I think it can be harmful to take frequent enemas and make them part of your life, because the colon was never meant to have things go up it, it's meant to have things go down. When someone is toxic, I use products that are colon cleansers that go in the mouth. There are people whose colons are practically paralyzed. It might be a neurological condition, or maybe they're paralyzed by long-term use of laxatives and enemas. But those aside, I tell people to keep their colon clean with the food they eat. Eating foods in their natural state is the best broom for their colon. Fiber, bentonite and psyllium husks are also very useful. I've never prescribed a laxative."

In addition, he recommends certain substances that, he says, are naturally detoxifying. "Anybody who has symptoms of toxemia: fatigue, bad breath, gasses from the body, or body odor. It's not natural to smell like a sewer, and some people do. I have them use spirulina, algae, chlorophyll and similar substances, because they're nutritious as well as detoxifying. They come in capsules, powders, and in liquids."

He is also an advocate of modified fasting: "When I graduated from medical school, I had a peptic ulcer and a gallbladder disturbance. I had to survive my internship, and none of the things I learned in school had worked. So I just closed myself up in my house and did nothing but sleep and drink bottled water, and at the end of five days or so, all my pain was gone." In the same manner, he later helped a relative: "He had a bleeding ulcer and had been taking aspirin for his back pain, and he ended up in a hospital and had to be given six pints of blood. I called him up and asked if he was ready to try my way. He got discharged from the hospital. I brought him back to my house and put him on nothing but water and grapefruit, and within a week he sounded so good his wife said, 'If you're going to stay out there on vacation, don't come back.' He went back, and he's never had another ulcer."

Some practitioners, we found, use more than just water when they recommend enemas. One personally uses a mixture containing castor oil, sesame oil, and licorice. He says it calms and cleanses the system. Another told us how he discovered an unusual mixture: "I was a medical student and working part-time at nights at a hospital. I had a patient who suffered with terrible constipation. The man had a chronic painful condition for which a doctor had given him large amounts of codeine, which was constipating him. So the doctor told me to give him a soap-suds enema. I tried it, and nothing much happened. Then the patient said, 'It won't work. Use equal parts whole milk and molasses.' It was amazing. I used a pint of milk and a pint of molasses, and he got a complete emptying of the large colon, with relative freedom from pain. I never found anything that works as well."

A Santa Monica physician told us he uses a variety of detox programs: "I put different kinds of people on cleansers depending on how I want to affect them. Sometimes it'll be juices, a colon cleanser, colonics, or it might just be changing their diets for a while. It depends on the complaints and on whether they need building, normalizing, or cleansing. If someone is depleted, I don't tend to fast or cleanse them. I try to build them up so they have the power to cleanse themselves. Basically, I don't try extraordinary measures unless we have an extraordinary situation."

He told us about one cleansing procedure that he recommends especially to women who want to get pregnant but have been exposed to toxins such as pesticides or have a history of drug abuse. "It involves three- to five-hour sessions daily. It's basically vitamins, minerals, salt tablets, potassium, homeopathic cell salts, oil and niacin, in addition to exercise and saunas. This is a way of getting fat-soluble residues out of fat cells, which include our brains and our livers. I give niacin, which breaks down fat cells, and the fat cells then release their toxins. This is followed by a sauna. You may also have to replenish the oil to the fat cells."

A San Diego physician told us, "I use detox procedures when

people are eating pretty bad diets and look like they need to lose weight. I put people on elimination diets as opposed to fasting. I use a protein powder that's hypo-allergenic and doesn't have the chemicals or other junk that some of the other mixtures have. Or I put them on what's called a cave man diet, which is basically vegetables and rice, and if they need protein, fish. This may last for one or two weeks. Depending on what we're trying to do, I might also have them eat raw vegetables, plus the protein powder so they're not wasting protein."

He told us of a gout patient he treated this way: "He had what looked like a pseudo-gout, which is basically hot, inflamed joints, mainly in the foot and the ankle. This can be pretty nasty. However, the blood test didn't confirm it was gout. We put him on an elimination diet, and in five or six days he was completely asymptomatic. Then I checked to see whether a food sensitivity was triggering the problem. I brought back the foods one at a time and looked for a reaction. It turned out that when he introduced orange juice, all of the symptoms returned overnight. He had hot, inflamed joints. There is some pretty hard evidence that even rheumatoid arthritis can be triggered by food allergies."

A Malibu doctor told us that she has used a combination of fasting and herbal preparations to cure patients with gallstones: "A gallbladder attack is one of the most excruciating pains you'll ever feel. The bile duct is one of the strongest muscles in the body, and when this nasty stone gets caught in it, most people feel as if somebody's stabbing them through the back with a knife. Most of them end up in surgery. But why does everybody who has their first, or even second, gallbladder attack have to have their gallbladder out? There are fasting programs using olive oil and garlic that help people eliminate gallstones. Many people have gallstones without symptoms.

"I never make anybody stop eating. What I do is ask them to be vegetarian for a week, along with herbal and fiber preparations. They ingest olive oil throughout the week, with a massive dose at the end. Olive oil is a liver cleanser. When you have grease, you don't get rid of it with water, you get rid of it with something that's a solvent. Olive oil works like a solvent. A massive amount causes the liver and the gallbladder to start releasing gallstones, and patients become much healthier."

Finally, a physician who ran a spa where cleansing fasts are featured: "The fasts average about two weeks—half the time fasting and half coming off the fast. We determine day by day whether they will have water or juice, or whether they're having vegetables or fruits. We've seen a number of people with supposedly incurable illnesses get well.

"One patient came to us because of extreme pain in the back of her head and severe neck tension. She could hardly move her shoulders, they were so stiff. Then she developed a whole series of skin cancers. She had so many the dermatologists were having a field day with her. She went through our fast, and her neck became mobile, she went back to playing golf, which she hadn't played for years, and the skin lesions that had developed into cancer just dropped off naturally."

NUTRITIONAL WELLNESS

It seems ironic that our day-to-day activities, the things we do for basic survival, should be so routinely overlooked by medical science. The things we eat and drink, how we exercise, the way we earn our livings, the air we breathe—what could be more fundamental to our health? Yet, historically, they have been relatively absent from scientific scrutiny. While nutrition was always central to other medical traditions, it was not considered as significant in the West until the 1920s, when vitamin deficiencies were scientifically proven to cause diseases like scurvy and beriberi and foods became specifically linked to the cause and treatment of disease. Even then, not much more was done, aside from epidemiological studies of the effects of diet on the health of large populations, until the correlations between diet and metabolic and cardiovascular diseases were found.

There were, of course, always a surfeit of competing theories and enough speculation, old wives' tales, and fads to keep purveyors of nutritional remedies in business. But it seems that the position of scientific medicine has basically been that eating is something we do to survive, and as long we eat a sensible, balanced diet we needn't peer any deeper into our larder for the causes and cures of disease.

Yet, as our interviews suggest, there are always those who believe that something as fundamental as food should not be treated lightly in the ongoing search for better health. With more and more emphasis on disease prevention and wellness, and with the limitless range of nutritional choice available to Americans, it seems inevitable that scientists will study more closely the relationships between specific foods and diseases. Ultimately, we will be able to separate speculation from fact and perhaps return to Hippocrates' injunction to regard our foods as our remedies.

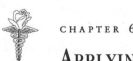
APPLYING HANDS-ON TREATMENT

Throughout the history of medicine there has been a wide variety of views regarding the optimal distance between the healer and the patient. At one extreme it is held that direct touch is essential for effecting a cure, while at the other, touching the patient seems anathema at worst or useless at best. In the first category are techniques ranging from the traditional laying on of hands to the systematic manipulation of the body. The hands-off family includes some religious or occult practitioners who reputedly invoke spiritual or energy forces without going near, or even seeing, the afflicted person. It could also include those physicians who diagnose and prescribe by telephone.

While modern medicine is often considered impersonal because of its technological emphasis, it has also seen a revival of the belief that physical contact plays a role in healing. For many years doctors have referred patients with musculoskeletal problems to physical therapists for rehabilitation. However, massage, manipulation, and relaxation techniques are now also commonly used, and innovative practices such as Reichian therapy, rolfing, and Alexander technique, in addition to other forms of what is loosely called "body work," are increasingly being employed. In addition, perhaps because of the inroads made by psychology, as well as voluminous accounts of childhood afflictions caused by the deprivation of human touch, doctors in recent years have been exhorted to provide more tender loving care (TLC)— including, when appropriate, the comforting touch of a hand.

Offshoots of modern medicine have also developed systems that entail touching, not for its own sake, but as a means of altering the structure of the body to cure disease. Chiropractic and osteopathy developed out of a belief that the human body requires readjustment not only because of traumas but also because of the inevitable consequences of two historical developments: the evolution of our species into upright, bipedal creatures whose organs are rearranged by gravity; and the ravages of industrial civilization, which places bodies designed for vigorous use into desk chairs, automobiles, and work conditions requiring ongoing distortions of posture. Both schools contend that structural misalignments create functional disorders by impeding nerve conduction, circulation, digestion, and other processes on whose integrity our health depends. Although chiropractic treatment has a wide public following, it has never been embraced by mainstream medicine, whereas osteopathic physicians (D.O.s) have, within recent years, been afforded the same privileges as medical doctors (M.D.s).

In this chapter, physicians discuss the use of unusual hands-on treatments that they picked up from informal sources. These range from manipulative techniques borrowed from chiropractors and osteopaths to the use of "healing energy" through touch. We also include unusual examples of another, related tradition: the direct application of various devices to the patient's body.

MANIPULATION

A New York physician told us that he had heard so many enthusiastic reports about chiropractic adjustments from patients that he ultimately sought training himself: "To me, the best treatment is the one with the best outcome. So if patients tell me they got better because of chiropractic treatment, I assume they mean it. I met some chiropractors who showed me what they did and let me observe firsthand, and I became convinced that patients were being helped. How long the improvement lasted varied with the chiropractor, the disease, and other factors, but the method had been proven to my satisfaction. I learned the techniques from my friends.

"I used it for back pain, obviously, and also for other problems when careful examination suggested it might be a good adjunctive treatment. Let me give you an example. I've treated several women for dysmenorrhea—painful menstruation. Chiropractic theory holds that a lot of that pain is due to congestion caused by blockages in the spine. Some disruption in the flow of cerebro-spinal fluid in that area causes disturbance in nerve conduction, affecting the nerves that supply the blood vessels, resulting in pain. That is the causal chain, theoretically, and if it's true, then the patient should feel better with chiropractic manipulation. If there were no underlying disease for which manipulation was contraindicated, I would use it, and it was surprising how well functional dysmenorrhea and other disturbances were improved by these treatments. If it were just a placebo, I wouldn't expect the improvement to last as long. I'm sure many patients would have gotten better if I hadn't done it, but I don't think they would have gotten better as fast."

We asked how his patients responded to receiving such unusual treatment: "People are actually a lot more liberal about these things than the doctors. Doctors treat chiropractors like they're charlatans, but patients know better. They just want to get help."

A pain specialist with a practice outside Los Angeles told us how he got interested in another form of manipulation: "I have back pain myself, and I noticed that when I bend over, I come up and curve to the side. I can't stand up straight. Once I was standing in front of the mirror and decided to move myself straight and wiggle my pelvis around. I just jerked myself around to see what would happen, and something popped. Something went boop! and I was straight again and didn't have any pain. I was just playing. I didn't know what I was doing. So I started investigating it and took some courses on mobilization of the spine.

"The particular type of mobilization I use is different from chiropractic, which has to do with high-velocity manipulation, where you move a joint through a short, hard, controlled jerk. With the mobilization I do, you use the body to move the joint. You hold a patient in a particular position, have him contract his muscles against you for a couple of seconds, have him relax, and then move the joint into the position you want it to go. Then you have him contract against you and move the joint again. I find it very useful, particularly for the spine. I had a couple of patients with neck pain who markedly improved with this treatment."

In discussing his sub-specialty, physical medicine, a San Diego physician told us about a method called SOT, for sacral occipital technique: "I was exposed to it when I had back pain. I was treating it with bed rest and pain medication when this friend of mine, a chiropractor, said, 'Why not come in and see me?' so I figured, 'Why not?' He gave me two treatments, and the results were dramatically effective. I realized that this is something that works. I didn't have to take any drugs, and the treatment was very gentle. It changed my whole opinion of the chiropractic profession. I had always been skeptical and often wondered if the effects were just basically psychological, but it was effective for me."

He took some seminars and incorporated SOT into his practice: "I use a procedure called blocking, where we place specially shaped wedges under the pelvis and hips. It's designed to take the contortion out of the dura, which is the membrane surrounding the spinal cord. Once we make the diagnosis, we assign the patient to one or more categories, then the blocks are placed in a certain position, at a certain angle, and the patient is tested.

"You change the position of the blocks until the testing indicates that they're properly placed. For one problem you might leave the patient there for thirty to sixty seconds, for others you might leave them for six minutes or more. Then you adjust the patient to see whether or not the placement of the blocks has strengthened the affected area and corrected the leg length difference. Then you do additional maneuvers that release the muscles in spasm. I don't do any bone adjustments. If the muscle is in spasm, I'll release the muscle with manipulation. If there's a tendon out of place, I'll return the tendon to its normal position. There's a variety of maneuvers for the neck and back, but, in many cases of lower back pain, blocking alone often relieves the pain."

A Malibu general practitioner spoke of an unusual osteopathic technique called cranial sacral manipulation: "It involves all the bones in the body, including those in the head. In a healthy person, the cranial bones move in a rhythmic fashion about ten or twelve times a minute. If there's an area where the bones are not moving freely, you simply restore mobility by altering the flow of cerebro-spinal fluid, lymphatic fluid, and blood. The procedure has been around for about fifty years, but it was only in the last ten or twenty years that some of the osteopathic schools decided to teach it. It's very subtle."

He said he uses the technique with newborns. "For example, there's a condition called pyloric stenosis, which is normally treated with surgery. It involves a spasm of the pyloric muscle at the bottom of the stomach, causing the baby to have projectile vomiting. In surgery, they actually cut through the muscle. In my experience, this condition is often simply due to pressure on a very sensitive nerve at the base of the skull. Along with the tremendous forces that are present during the birth process, this can cause the bones at the base of the skull to be compressed. By very gently opening up the area, a lot of these symptoms totally disappear."

We asked about the use of the technique on adults: "One memorable patient was a young woman who had been in an auto accident. Her main complaints were headaches and dizziness. She had seen ear, nose, and throat specialists and several neurologists. But after a cranial sacral treatment, the dizziness was totally gone and she had no more headaches. The manipulation is very gentle. You're simply working with the forces present in the body."

A family physician in Boston told us about an osteopathic technique she learned from a friend: "It's a trigger release technique. It entails finding a very tender trigger point in the muscles of the upper back and, while putting pressure on that point, moving the arm and shoulder until the tenderness is relieved. Then you hold that position for a certain amount of time. You apply it when somebody has pain in the upper back. This is not found in any standard repertoire or in postgraduate education. But I've found it effective on myself, so I'm convinced that it works. Without it, I would have used heating pads and stretching exercises or perhaps anti-inflammatory drugs."

BODY WORK

Particularly in California, a number of systematic variations on massage and body movement that fall under the general rubric of "body work" have gained popularity. Several of our respondents said they occasionally refer patients to credentialed practitioners of these techniques, and two even provided office space for them. One family practitioner in Los Angeles was particularly fond of such procedures. We'll let him speak for the rest:

"I'm a big believer in body work. I have a network of people who do rolfing, Alexander technique, Feldenkrais, shiatsu, and Reichian therapy. I send patients to them all the time—people with chronic tension, where certain muscle groups in the neck and back and shoulders are knotted up like rocks and they have do some deep tissue work to loosen them up, or people with back, neck, or facial pain, or sciatica. I have learned which of these techniques work best with different problems. I've had people who would otherwise be on pain medication or be told they need surgery, and if they have the patience to work with a technician over time, they usually get better. Not always, of course. Some cases are too advanced, but most patients can be helped with body work if they cooperate.

"I also use massage or body work for stress reduction. The musculature has a kind of memory that embodies the tension. If someone has emotional upsets or constant pressures, or even deep-rooted childhood traumas, they get deposited somewhere in the body or the nervous system and stay there and may throw other organs and systems off balance. Some deep massage, structural realignment, and work on the connective tissue can relieve a lot of that tension and get the system working properly. However, it's not just for pain or obvious pressure. It's to get the blood and other fluids circulating properly, because circulation in parts of the body can become stagnant. I've had a lot of success with arthritis and stress-related disorders, such as ulcers, hypertension, headaches, and digestive problems. I can get these patients off their medication if they see a body worker regularly.

"I myself was trained in reflexology, and I offer that to some of my patients if they're open to it. Almost any disorder can be helped with it. There are certain points on the feet that are like reflex buttons that are connected to different parts of the body. The body is all wired together electrically. If you massage these points in a certain way, they stimulate the corresponding parts and free up the healing forces, so the body can cure itself. For example, there are points on the feet that connect to the throat. If you massage them, you can help someone who has a sore throat. Someone who is constipated can be helped by working on those points connected to the colon."

THE TOUCH OF YOUR HANDS

Several doctors told us that they make a point of simply touching their patients, particularly in areas where there is pain. In most cases this is done simply as a gesture of comfort and reassurance, which they believe to be important in its own right. But a few of our respondents took touching a step further. They felt that there might be a genuine value in the notion of "laying on of hands," and they attributed some degree of healing power to their own touch. Here is a Southern California doctor with an otherwise traditional family practice:

"I discovered at one point that I had some healing ability. As a child, I felt I was clairaudient and could hear voices within me. Some years ago I was doing a process called rebirthing, and I noticed that my hands felt extremely hot. When I went to write about my observations, I could sense something coming through them. I decided to just relax and go with it, and what came out were messages to me. I was very much in turmoil at the time. My marriage was falling apart and I was very uncertain about going to medical school."

The experience led her to study with a purported healer: "I'd heard of her and wanted to find out what this healing business was about. People said that healing is an ability that everyone has and can learn to reinforce through experience. After I completed my medical training, I would sometimes use energy healing on patients, although I didn't tell them that was what I was doing. For example, a woman brought her boyfriend into my office. He had vomiting attacks and severe abdominal pain. I put him in the hospital and called a surgeon. That night I went to see him. He was retching so bad they couldn't give him medication. Finally, I put my hand on his abdomen, started running energy, and I got him calmed down. When I went in to see him later on, he said, 'I felt what you were doing the other day, and it really helped.' They never did find out what was wrong with him. I'm convinced it was an emotional reaction to something and that my touch calmed him down.

"I don't do that normally. I've been holding back because I've been afraid of people's reactions. Sometimes, when I have a patient on the examining table and he's talking to me, I put my hands on him. He doesn't know what's going on. I did it on my son, too. Once he had a bad fever and flu symptoms, and I didn't have any antibiotics in the house, so I put my hands on him, and he was fine. I know I have a lot of energy running through my body. Part of what I've learned is that the more work I do on myself, the more I open my heart and let go of my blocks, the more energy I can give to my patients."

A family physician in Colorado told us this remarkable personal story: "I was in my late thirties and had reached all my lifetime goals. Yet, I found to my dismay that I was dissatisfied. It occurred to me that although I had heard the word 'spirit' all my life, I knew virtually nothing about the spiritual component of human health. At the same time, I was feeling increasing frustration with conventional medicine's inability to successfully treat chronic diseases.

"It was then that I made the first of five trips to Fiji, where I encountered the most spiritual, loving, and balanced people I had ever met. They seemed to have a personal relationship with God, and, as a group, were extremely healthy and happy. Traditional Fijian medicine uses little more than prayer, touch, herbs, and plants. That trip was the inspiration and the catalyst I needed to commit to my own spiritual journey."

Back home, he studied with a mystic theologian: "After I had completed one year of study, he said to me, 'You have the most powerful healing touch I've ever felt.' I was stunned. I wasn't sure what to make of his words, but it did occur to me that such a gift could be a pretty handy tool for a doctor. It certainly worked well for the Fijians. He told me the only way to develop the full potential of a healing touch was to use it as much as possible. He said the ability is a gift, that the healer is a channel for God's energy, and that the essence of this energy is love.

"I unofficially began a new career as a spiritual healer. My first patient was a friend who had fractured a femur and was hospitalized. He was in considerable post-op pain after extensive surgery. I treated him with touch, and within several hours he was pain-free without the use of narcotics. His orthopedist said that most patients require almost two weeks of narcotics following this surgery. He was out of the hospital in three days. Another friend was told that he needed surgery for a herniated disc. After a couple of my touch treatments, he, too, was pain-free and has never had any further back problems.

"I spent a month in Fiji, where I saw eleven patients, beginning with a man who had an immobile shoulder. All of them got better following one touch treatment. The day before I left I was asked to treat a seventy-two-year-old man with glaucoma who had been totally blind for five years. He had been to the Western doctors in the capital city, only to be told that nothing more could be done for him. I gave him a twenty-minute treatment and returned the next morning on my way to the airport. I asked if there had been any change. He said, 'Yes, I can now see all of my fingers when I hold my hands in front of my face.'

"I was moved to tears of joy, overwhelmed with awe at the power of God, and I knew I would never practice medicine as I had before. Since then, I've combined my own self-healing journey with a holistic practice. I continue to use some touch healing, but because the concept is so alien to our cultural belief system, the results are not quite as consistent or dramatic as they were in Fiji."

Here is a story from a veteran doctor who availed himself of a healer for his own medical problem: "I did a study of healers because I had a patient who teaches it and she said anyone can learn to do it. She belonged to a group of six or seven healers who met in West Los Angeles. At that time, I had problems with leg pains. I went to one healer, who accomplished nothing. That same evening, I went to another woman who said, 'Don't tell me what's wrong with you. Just lie down.' She put her hands over my body. When she touched me, I thought it was diathermy; it was that hot. She said, 'Oh, my, you have bad problems with your legs and back, don't you? I'll take care of it.'

"Well, after one treatment the pain went away. I saw her about once every six months when it would recur. Then I lost track of her, and I did not have the same results with the other healers, so I ended up using medication. Healers are fascinating. But, unfortunately, those I have met since then have been ineffectual. I'm still looking, though. I want to check them out because healing touch is a whole area that should be explored systematically."

INSCRUTABLE TOUCH

A few doctors told us about hands-on techniques derived from China. One we heard about several times was acupressure, which is finger pressure applied to traditional acupuncture points in lieu of needles. Here is a story of role reversal from a Los Angeles G.P.:

"I broke my shoulder and was working with my arm in a splint. Toward the end of the day I saw a patient whom I'd been seeing for some time. After I finished, she said, 'You look like you're in a lot of pain. Why don't you let me do some acupressure on you?' And I thought, 'I don't need this. Let me go home and take a pain pill.' But she was persistent and wanted to be helpful, so I said, 'Why not? What could it hurt?'

"She had me repeat after her some kind of incantations, a mantra, while she used her knuckles to exert pressure on my shoulders, chest, back, and neck. It went on for some time and was painful, but about two hours later, I felt greatly relieved of my discomfort. I was impressed and sorry that I did not learn more about it, but I was rather staid and orthodox in my medical outlook then." At the time, he said, he felt it inappropriate to recommend something as unconventional as acupressure to patients just because it worked for him. Eventually, however, he began to recommend the procedure.

An internist from San Francisco told us an amusing acupressure story: "I've had a lot of patients who respond to acupressure. If you just teach people a few pressure points, they can apply it themselves; it can be very successful. There's one Jewish grandmother type who had headaches and sinus trouble. I taught her the points for treating those conditions. It was very significant because it meant that she could do something for herself to help alleviate a problem that had been causing her pain and suffering for years. Anyway, it cleared up significantly, and she started making other changes in her life because she felt so much better. Soon, she'd lost twenty pounds. One day she came in and confided in me that her husband was exhausted: she'd been chasing him around the house because she had so much sexual energy."

A physician who studied with a Taoist master told us about a procedure called *chi lei jong:* "It's a technique of energy transformation in the organs. It's basically a form of massage of the abdomen. It's not aimed at a particular complaint, but at moving energy blockages from the abdominal organs and the musculature throughout the body. It redirects blood flow and lymphatic fluid."

He said that virtually every patient could benefit from the technique, but that he uses it mainly "with gastric ulcers, or when there is a consistent complaint of abdominal pain, without pathological findings. For example, one woman with irritable bowel syndrome had been treated by other physicians with medications, as well as with acupuncture and homeopathy. She was holding in a lot of anger and anxiety, and once the layers of energy had been unblocked, the irritable bowel syndrome went away.

"That patient would come in weekly, and I'd send her home with instructions on how to work on herself. It takes about five to ten treatments as a general rule. I tell patients to do it at least once a day, and each time they come in, I teach them a little more. It's essential that they realize that the healing comes from within them and not from me or from my wonderful hands.

"It's not just for abdominal problems. There was an older man in his eighties who complained of numbness in his leg, which I felt was due to an arterial spasm. There was not enough blood coming through to the leg. I worked on his abdomen and the arterial pulses in the leg, and I was able to redirect the blood flow. The procedure varies from patient to patient. There's a certain sequence you go through that's the same for everyone, but each patient has areas of specificity. It's actually time consuming. It's something you do if you are willing to spend the time."

As an extension of the use of hands, some doctors described techniques involving the use of special gadgets and devices. We begin with a relatively common procedure that has been inching closer to the mainstream over the past fifteen or twenty years, and then move on to more unusual devices.

One of our respondents was an early proponent of biofeedback, the process by which one learns to self-regulate bodily functions through feedback from monitoring devices: "In 1971, I had been in practice only a few months when a patient with severe anxiety disorder, who wasn't responding to any type of conventional treatment, came to see me. I didn't know what else to do for her. She was in agony and felt possessed by demonic forces which consumed her with horrible thoughts. She was hurting herself in attempting to get relief."

He decided to try a new technique he had seen demonstrated a few months earlier, using feedback on brain-wave patterns in an attempt to reduce anxiety: "The woman made a rather spectacular improvement. I was somewhat shocked because we had tried everything available to modern psychiatry with no success. She was connected to a machine that records changes in brain waves, indicated by different colored lights. All she had to do was follow the instructions. In the beginning, she was blank, worried, and preoccupied, but after a few sessions, she started to smile and even joked with us. The difference was undeniable. I was then able to lower her medication. Eventually, she only needed a small dose to allay the anxiety, and she was able to go out and get a job.

"I started using it in my private practice, not only with psychiatric patients but also those with pain syndromes, insomnia, and other conditions. I developed a psychodynamic approach, combining psychotherapeutic techniques with the physiological application of standard biofeedback. For example, I had no idea why one of my patients was having anxiety attacks, but I had noted that the minute she got anxious she would swing her foot. On this particular day she had been doing that continuously. So I hooked her up to a GSR, which measures skin conduction, and asked her to recall and talk about various people in her life. It turned out that what she *thought* made her anxious was not really the case. The GSR responded markedly when she talked about her mother, not when she spoke about her boyfriend, whom she said she felt anxious about. However, it turned out that she felt some guilt and fear about recently confronting her mother, who had a heart condition. She thought that confrontation might contribute to her mother's untimely death. She had no awareness that that had anything to do with her anxiety attacks."

A pain specialist in Los Angeles uses biofeedback at his clinic: "We use the simplest equipment. There are some sensors you put on the fingers and arms which read muscle tension. We use temperature biofeedback, which denotes the amount of blood flow in the peripheral tissue. It's a matter of using your mind to control the physiological basis of pain. The most common headache we see is the muscle contraction headache. We teach patients that at the first sign of a headache, they should do their biofeedback exercises. When the vasoconstriction phase starts, they can dilate the blood vessels in their brain by using our device. I have a lot of migraine patients who don't have to take any drugs at all. We also use it to control muscle spasm. Patients with Reynaud's disease can warm their ice cold hands and stop the stimulation that constricts the blood vessels."

The doctor said that he treated his own high blood pressure with biofeedback. "My forty-nine-year-old father had died in my arms of a coronary. So, when I developed hypertension and turned fifty, I was naturally frightened. I went on a diet and started exercising religiously, but I didn't want to take medication because of the side effects. So I did biofeedback. We were already using it with our pain patients, so

I hooked myself up and found I could really relax. After a couple of sessions, I could drop my blood pressure. I got my own unit to use at home, and I found I could bring my blood pressure down to normal and it would stay within an acceptable level."

A less well-known instrument was discussed by a doctor who used it in a drug detoxification program: "It's called 'transcranial electro-therapy.' It was designed to relax patients by synchronizing their brain waves, and, at the same time, possibly effecting the release of endorphins by applying minuscule alternating currents to the brain. We placed electrodes on the ear lobes and applied current through the skin. A very small electric current spreads into the cranial cavity. We used it for pain management, alcohol detoxification, and stress reduction. Essentially, the rationale is to stabilize the neuroelectric or neurochemical environment.

"We tried to help addicts get their fix, if you will, from electricity and acupuncture rather than from drugs. In addition, we gave them a great deal of nutritional support instead of medicine. The main objective was to help patients get through the more difficult periods of the withdrawal process."

One interesting, and controversial, use of technology that was discussed by two of the physicians we interviewed is a process called chelation. First, a Beverly Hills G.P. explains what it is: "Chelation therapy is a procedure for reducing arteriosclerosis by removing ionic calcium from the arteries themselves. Calcium is the mortar that holds arterial plaque in place, so getting rid of it is the first step in removing plaque—the fatty deposits that block the arteries. It works by infusing small amounts of a substance called disodium ethylene-diamine tetra-acetic acid (EDTA) into the bloodstream, which then binds to ionic calcium. That process is called chelation. It entails a painless, slow intravenous drip of EDTA solution over a three- or four-hour period. The patient, while seated, can read, talk, or even take a nap. The number of treatments depends on the condition."

He explained the origins of the therapy: "EDTA was originally used in the treatment of lead poisoning. You can remove lead from the blood and tissues with an intravenous infusion of EDTA. In the early fifties it was reported that some physicians using this treatment noticed that patients with lead poisoning who had arteriosclerosis showed marked improvement. This led to use with people who had had a heart attack, bypass surgery, or a stroke—all the signs of artery blockage. Some physicians even use it as a preventive procedure for high-risk patients. In my experience, chelation patients show noticeable effects of improved blood circulation: better exercise tolerance and kidney function, a reduction of angina, and even clearer thinking.

"It's very safe. In terms of complications, I believe that EDTA is safer than aspirin. I'm not aware of any fatalities connected with chelation. During the treatment, there might be a temporary lowering of blood sugar or blood pressure, or some cramping in the arms and legs, but these are easily controlled by adjusting the dosage. True, it has been a controversial treatment and the regulating agencies have been very skeptical of it. But, in my judgment, it's not only safe, but it should be regarded as a major advancement in the fight against heart disease."

A New York physician said he has used chelation with an estimated 2,500 patients: "We use a synthetic amino acid because it's so foreign the body rejects it, and it doesn't break down. Virtually one hundred percent of it is excreted from the body unchanged, except that in its course through the bloodstream it picks up divalent metal ions. We're talking about calcium, zinc, copper, lead, cadmium, and aluminum—some of those are toxic, while others are essential. We replace the ones we feel are essential. Chelation relieves a lot of the symptoms of atherosclerosis. Whether we actually *reverse* atherosclerosis has been the subject of a lot of discussion. I think that over time we actually do that. People certainly show dramatic improvement and that's what they come to me for."

As to skepticism, he pointed out that there were skeptics when the method was first used on lead poisoning: "It was immediately branded as worthless. People felt there was nothing you could do to get lead out of the body. They wouldn't even look at the test results that showed the lead being eliminated in the urine. But ultimately, cooler heads prevailed and they began using it to treat people with lead poisoning, who previously had had a totally hopeless prognosis.

"In the early days, chelation had some damaging side effects. Patients were incurring kidney damage because they were getting huge doses that we no longer think are safe. There was no way then to know what a safe dose was. We've greatly improved the therapeutic ratio, which refers to the number of people who have a therapeutic result without any adverse side effects."

One of the physicians who earlier described his adoption of chiropractic techniques told us of a second addition to his practice, which began when he discovered a machine called the electroacuscope: "I met a physical therapist in my office, who told me about an instrument he used to treat pain and was interested in using it with my patients. I'd heard of it because I'm a golfer and there were people like Jack Nicklaus who swore by it. So I said, 'Okay, I have a patient who's in agony with two broken ribs and can't roll over. See what you can do for him.'

"We treated the patient on a Thursday and Friday. Over the weekend, he had minimal pain and remained that way. I told the therapist, 'I don't know of any modality that will get rid of the pain from broken ribs.' He wasn't treating acupuncture sites or nerves. He was just treating the pain site. Since then, I've learned that the instrument can be valuable."

The doctor later took a training course, bought his own electroacuscope, and started using it in his practice along with a related machine: "They're called micro-current physical therapy instruments. They measure and correct areas of altered electrical activity in your tissues. If there is a disturbance in the normal impedance, the instrument will correct it. This is not metaphysical. Charged particles, ions, essential for cell maintenance and growth, normally enter and exit the cell. But with an injury or a disease process, the movement of these particles across the cell membrane is blocked, causing physical changes that can be detected and corrected.

"There are two brass-tipped electrodes about the size of large pins. One emits the current and the other picks it up. The instrument interprets any distortion as the signal passes through the tissue. You can also use it for diagnostic purposes. For example, when you place electrodes above and below the area of pain, you can get a digital readout. If there is evidence of a blockage, that's the place that needs treatment. If you put the electrodes on either side of an area where there is no problem, you should get a normal reading.

"It causes only a mild tingling sensation. The intensity of the treating current is designed to be strong enough to be able to pass through the tissue and reach the other electrode. One well-accepted theory on pain is that because of increased permeability of the cell membrane there is leakage of inflammatory substances in the interstitial environment. These stimulate the pain fibers in the area, and the brain interprets it as being painful. That's what makes it hurt. By treating the afflicted areas locally, you can seal off those membranes and normalize conductivity so that the nerve doesn't tell the brain that there is pain. Back spasms occur when the nerve passing to a muscle is irritated and sends a signal to the muscle to contract. So when we treat a patient with muscle spasm, we treat the nerve that's involved."

We asked if these machines were considered acceptable by his colleagues: "Doctors can accept using such instruments for the treatment of muscle spasms. That's not a big reach for the average physician. But what they have difficulty in accepting is that the same process is applicable to a wide variety of conditions. That's the exciting part. In the beginning I was just treating back pain and headaches. But I began to realize that once you accept the idea that an energy deficiency in the tissues can be corrected, it opens up entirely new possibilities for treatment.

"One exciting use is to stimulate acupuncture points. I use it on patients with injuries. For an injury to a calf muscle, I treat the muscle and nerve at the appropriate spinal cord level. For a patient with a headache, I'll treat acupuncture sites on the ear and face.

"This technique is also very effective with skin problems. I get referrals from a vascular surgeon for patients with diabetic and arterial-insufficiency ulcers of the skin. These conditions respond very well to electrical stimulation, and sometimes chronic ulcers heal in a week or two. I apply it to either side of the ulcers. Stimulation is passed across the ulcer bed and along the acupuncture meridian running through the ulcer. Normally, these kinds of ulcers are treated with dressings, whirlpool treatment, medication, and surgery. I had a patient last year with an ulcer the size of a half-dollar. He had it for over a year and was being treated at a hospital with dressings and whirlpool, and it wasn't improving. We treated him intensively. Twice a day the first week, then daily for the next two weeks, then every other day. After eight weeks, it appeared to be totally healed, and since that time, it hasn't broken down. Not only is the ulcer healed but the energy is normalized throughout that area so the skin doesn't break down as easily. Now the skin is tougher, it looks better, and the patient is grateful.

"I've had at least four or five patients in the last two years who canceled scheduled surgery. For example, one patient was scheduled to have surgery for carpal tunnel syndrome, which is a compression of the median nerve in the wrist. The patient got a few treatments and recovered completely. Another patient with a herniated disk had weakness in his arm along with numbness and severe radiating pains. He made about an eighty percent recovery. He still has some symptoms, but the pain is minimal. We saved him an operation. Also, he has no surgical scars or complications. The insurance company saved a lot of money."

Another one of our respondents, a Santa Monica G.P., spoke enthusiastically about the myopulse, which she called a sister machine to the acuscope: "I'm not using it on patients yet. I'm trying it out on myself and my family, specifically for the small muscles of the face. Because there are a lot of acupuncture points on the face, it stimulates the meridians for the lungs, liver, kidneys, ovaries, intestines, and other organs. A colleague has had good results with chronic fatigue syndrome, and it's proven effective for muscle pains and injuries. The frequency wave on the myoscope is different from that of the acuscope. It's more effective in treating muscles.

We asked for an example of the machine's use: "I pulled a muscle in my neck and couldn't move my head. I woke up that way and went to work, like an idiot, but I couldn't function. So I consulted a colleague who put a myoscope probe directly on the area, in my ear, and on an acupuncture point. I had no other treatment. Four hours later I had full mobility and no pain at all. A friend of mine had a pelvic infection and had been on a lot of antibiotics for several weeks. I used a vaginal probe and got rid of all the pain."

Her explanation for why such machines work was nonspecific: "It works because we are not just chemical but electrical beings. There's an electrical system in the body, and when there's an injury, inflammation, or damage, the electrical field in that area is disturbed. Basically, when you use the proper frequency, the chemical activity changes, and the electrical balance is restored."

THE COMMON TOUCH

A few years ago, the newspapers reported, with considerable fanfare, the results of a controlled study that demonstrated that hospitalized patients who were touched on a regular basis had a significantly better recovery rate than those for whom touch was withheld. This struck many observers as far too obvious to justify the research dollars. But, as I mentioned in the context of nutrition, the obvious is sometimes the last place science looks. In the late nineteenth century, it took Edward Livingston Trudeau many years to convince people that fresh air could be a vital element in the treatment of tuberculosis. Quite possibly, something as simple as the human touch might soon be regarded as medically indispensable. As the boundaries of mainstream medicine inevitably expand, we might begin to take it literally when someone says of his doctor, "I'm in good hands."

CHAPTER 7

MAKING USE OF
OTHER MEDICAL TRADITIONS

In recent years, thanks to cultural diffusion, enhanced communication, and the historical forces described in chapter one, American physicians have become increasingly aware of sophisticated systems of medicine that are fundamentally different from their own. Many of the doctors we interviewed have incorporated elements of such systems into their repertoire of nostrums, while a few now specialize in them and have transformed their practices entirely. The systems in question are principally Chinese medicine, the Ayurvedic system of India, and homeopathy, which has had a wide following in Europe and is enjoying a revival in the U.S., where it had been popular until early this century.

CHINESE MEDICINE

The first few excerpts concern the ancient Chinese art of acupuncture. When it became better known to Western physicians in the 1970s, acupuncture was highly controversial. The idea of effecting cures by inserting needles into points on the skin was, naturally, greeted with skepticism. Theoretically, stimulating specific acupuncture points in that manner activates pathways called meridians, along which energy is directed to the various organs. The process is said to facilitate the body's natural healing mechanisms. Since the existence of such meridians was never actually established anatomically, the purported effects of acupuncture were dismissed as artifacts of suggestion and belief. Nevertheless, acupuncture's apparent efficacy as a pain reliever and an anesthetic sparked considerable interest. Gradually some insurance carriers began to cover acupuncture treatment for certain conditions, and scores of Western physicians began to acquire specialized training in the practice.

A specialist in physical medicine and rehabilitation told us he uses acupuncture along with Western procedures in treating pain. "I was attracted to acupuncture because it's been used for thousands of years. The Chinese developed a system to treat a lot of chronic diseases and intractable pain problems that are still treated less effectively today by traditional Western medicine. I've had success with whiplash problems, for example. People had been going to therapy for several years but still had a lot of neck and shoulder pain radiating out to the arms. They had to constantly take medication, but after several acupuncture treatments, they improved significantly.

"I've also had success using acupuncture for diabetic peripheral neuropathy pain. People with diabetes sometimes get pain in their hands and feet, which often does not respond to conventional pain medicine. Also frozen shoulder. The capsule around the shoulder joint gets stuck together and patients have trouble moving their shoulders. You can treat the pain and get them moving better with acupuncture."

A number of doctors we interviewed have carried their interest in acupuncture beyond the treatment room. Take, for example, this physician/researcher who had what he terms a "big shift" in his thinking in the early seventies when he studied pain mechanisms: "There was a lot of controversy about acupuncture at that time. Doctors assumed that the effects were purely psychological. However, I had a medical student of Chinese descent whose family had done acupuncture in Asia, and he wanted to research it. He worked on his own, sometimes till the wee hours of the morning. He started to get interesting results and found he could actually block the neural pain messages in animals with acupuncture. We continued to collect the data, but didn't publish it because we didn't know what the hell it meant. We didn't think anybody would believe us anyway.

"Our data suggested that the results could be due to something like endorphins [morphine-like molecules that the brain produces to counteract pain]. We tested the hypothesis in our animals and discovered that acupuncture does stimulate endorphin production. That changed my life. We traveled all over Asia visiting clinics and hospitals, and we saw many remarkable things."

Eventually, the doctor developed an electrical machine that enables practitioners to do acupuncture without needles. "You put an electrode pad on the skin and stimulate the nerves underneath. The advantage over needles is that patients can treat themselves at home. I think daily treatment is very important for chronic conditions because the effects are cumulative. Acupuncture, as it's practiced in the Western world, once or twice a week, is not the correct way. Also, Western M.D.s learn how to use the needles in only a few weekend courses, but it actually takes years of experience to do it right. There's supposed to be an aching sensation in the acupuncture site called *de qi*. With the needle, you have to hit the point spot-on. You have to get the right depth and angle, and you have to twirl the needle correctly so you hurt the patient just a little bit but not too much. Most clinicians in the West are afraid to hurt their patients, thinking they won't come back. As a result, the treatment is not properly given.

"The machine makes it much easier to learn and administer. The pad covers a wide area. The electrical charge activates an entire region, and the nerve picks it up. So, for pain, you only need to know a couple of dozen points. Also, the patients can turn the dial themselves, so they learn to apply just the right amount of current.

"We've treated ten thousand patients and have three double-blind control studies. What's really surprising is not only that their pain goes away but that they're apparently cured. We don't fully understand that. We do a follow-up eight months later, and their pain hasn't come back. With other procedures, the pain comes back. It's what the Chinese have been saying all along, but nobody believed them.

"I think medicine is very tunnel-visioned. There isn't one treatment, one magic potion for everything. Medicine is an art and an empirical process. A good doctor uses the best of everything."

VARIATIONS ON THE THEME

A number of physicians have adopted unusual variations of acupuncture. This San Diego doctor told us about a system that he learned in England: "It's called five-element acupuncture. The idea is to view symptoms as reflections of an underlying energy imbalance in one of five elements which are analogous to wood, water, fire, earth, and metal. In our diagnosis, we divide diseases into physical, mental, and spiritual levels within each of the five elements. So there are physical manifestations of the elements, emotional manifestations, and behavioral or lifestyle manifestations. It's a very helpful matrix to use to evaluate people in order to plan how to approach their problems."

We asked how the treatments themselves differ from what we normally associate with acupuncture. "The technique is a bit different," the doctor replied. "We use very minimal stimulation of the points and we usually don't leave the needles in. Our intention is to connect to what's called the spirit of the point. The idea is to use the points to redefine the person and help him evolve into a healthier state. If you can match the energy of the point and the situation, some pretty remarkable things happen. For example, one point on the lung meridian is called the Very Great Abyss. It is a metaphor for patients who feel depressed, hopeless, and in the pits."

The doctor said he was drawn to this system when he heard a lecture about it in the early 1970s. Over time, he has added elements of his own to five-element acupuncture. "I've added some very specific treatments for pain. Acupuncture has many styles to it. You open up the door of acupuncture, and there is a variety of directions you can go in. With some disorders you can have a formula, but with difficult conditions almost every treatment is different."

He described some of his more memorable cases: "There have been some miraculous one-treatment effects. One woman had tic douloureux, which is trigeminal neuralgia—severe, intractable pain in the face, around the jaw muscles. She had been through everything. They were at the point of cutting the nerve, which is what they do in a extreme situation. I treated one acupuncture point, and it went away after the first treatment. The point was Gall Bladder One, an entry-point meridian that starts in the face. It was astonishing.

"Then there was an executive who had suprascapular neuritis, with constant pain above the shoulder and into the neck. It was incapacitating enough to prevent her from traveling. She'd had it for three years and had had no results with physical therapy. I treated her two or three times with appropriate acupuncture points, and she had an eighty to ninety percent clearance."

A physician who now practices in Los Angeles uses another variation: "It's based on Korean acupuncture, in which the hand is used exclusively instead of the whole body. Magnets are put on acupuncture points on the hands. They create an ionic flow within the body, which opens up the different channels. You tape them on a point for as little as twenty minutes or as long as twenty-four hours. It's less painful to the patient and very effective. I had a woman recently with post-herapeutic neuralgia. She had had chronic pain between the ribs caused by a viral infection, and she'd been treated with pain killers for twenty-three years. A few treatments, and she was free of pain."

NEEDLES AND HERBS

The Chinese view disease as a sign of an imbalance between yin, which is associated with the material properties of the body, and yang, which is said to be the energy that drives physical processes. Treatment is designed to re-establish that balance. Typically, this entails a combination of acupuncture and herbal prescriptions from the complex Chinese pharmacopoaia. One physician-turned-acupuncture-specialist explained this in the context of Chinese medical history: "What's coming out of China now is called traditional Chinese medicine, but its tradition is only about thirty years old. It was put together by Mao in response to the need for generalized health care. He organized the remaining acupuncturists and herbalists in China into schools of traditional Chinese medicine. Over the course of years, they distilled the traditional knowledge and declared one philosophy to be the traditional approach to Chinese medicine. In that particular philosophy, acupuncture is used as a backup to herbal prescriptions.

"There are all sorts of sophisticated models that explain disease. In any of these models, one can support using acupuncture with herbs. For example, herbal preparations can be useful as a pharmacological substrate to tone or calm the system, or to balance the strengths and weaknesses, excesses and deficiencies of the organs. The effect of acupuncture lasts longer if you give an herbal formula that targets specific organs. Generally, I'll use an herbal preparation if the problem is old or chronic and the vitality of the patient is diminished. The herbal remedies build up the patient's strength and ability to respond.

"About thirty percent of my practice deals with pain as the primary problem. I also get people who feel limited in what they can do because they have frequent colds, bronchitis that persists for months, a nervous stomach that acts up more than is convenient, or diarrhea. In orthodox medicine those conditions would be considered relatively minor functional complaints. Those symptoms identify the weak link in the patient's makeup, and quite often they predispose the patient to more serious problems.

"Take bronchitis, for example. If it's acute, you can get a rapid response. It is completely possible that one or two acupuncture treatments will open up the lungs and help the body rally to resolve the condition. If it's a recurrent bronchitis, then it takes a little bit longer to treat. You need to deal with the immediate symptoms and then address the entire composition of the patient and work to build up any particular system that is weak. If it has set in and become chronic, the effect of acupuncture can be enhanced by the use of herbs to clear the phlegm from the patient's chest, to calm the dry cough, or tone the energy of their lungs."

When we asked him to be specific regarding the Chinese herbs he would use for different conditions, he declined: "I'm not going to do that. If one makes any prescription, be it acupuncture or herb, it is based on the individual patient. And, since we don't have a patient here, I can't prescribe."

One physician we interviewed has used acupuncture and Chinese herbs in a substance-abuse clinic with what he says is considerable success: "The counselors in our program learned about acupuncture for helping drug abuse withdrawal, so they invited some specialists in to give a demonstration. I didn't think it would work. But it became obvious that the patients benefited and that they liked it. We started using acupuncture on a pilot basis and gradually learned what points to use and how to do it correctly. It seems to control withdrawal symptoms and craving. I think it has a balancing effect on the auto-nomic nervous system."

With respect to the use of Chinese herbs, he said: "We kept modifying the formulas and trying them out with different patients, and that worked out quite well. We used herbs to relax substance abusers."

Another physician claimed to have used Chinese medicine to treat AIDS patients: "AIDS is a new disease, but the patterns of imbalance have been recognized for thousands of years in the Chinese tradition. Chinese medical books describe ways to improve immune function. The nature of the disease and the fact that a lot of other treatments are being used simultaneously makes it hard to assess exactly how well the Chinese medicine is working, but I think acupuncture and herbs provide a good deal of relief from AIDS symptoms. Many patients report an improved sense of well-being, and some have gained weight and returned to work."

INDIAN TRADITIONS

The other products of Asia that have met with some favor in the West stem from the ancient traditions of India. The best known of these imports is hatha yoga, the system of stretches, postures, and breathing exercises widely practiced for fitness and relaxation. However, it has also attracted some interest in the treatment of disease, especially musculoskeletal disorders. Several of our doctors said they recommend yoga for back and neck pain, as well as conditions associated with stress. This family physician uses it extensively:

"For example, a man came to me who had fallen on a plate-glass table and incurred serious back strain. He was getting some physical therapy and massage, but wasn't showing any improvement. I sent him to a yoga class, and he got considerable relief from his pain, and it made his other physical therapies more effective."

The doctor said she also prescribes yogic breathing exercises: "Oxygen is the common denominator of all energy transformation. Without oxygen everything slows down and the whole system becomes sluggish.

"I teach my patients to breathe correctly. Most of us do what I call 'survival breathing.' We breathe with half or less of our chests, and the muscles that actually do the deep breathing get lazy and resistant. I teach people to breathe completely and to use four or five deep breaths to center themselves and quiet themselves down. Relaxation is crucial in at least three quarters of the illness that I see."

She said she finds breathing exercises especially valuable for asthma patients: "Often asthmatics not only can't get enough oxygen but their breathing muscles are very tight. Deep-breathing exercises help them get more oxygen into their lungs. Our lungs are like balloons, and the bottom of our lungs is where fluid collects and bacteria thrive. I encourage patients to use that image of a balloon to help them fill their lungs completely. With patients who have great difficulty breathing deeply, I use medicines to get them started—bronchodilators to help relax the tubes that let oxygen in."

She added that one reason breathing exercise helps asthmatics is psychological: "It gives them a feeling of control. For some asthmatic patients, part of their problem is panic and a sense of being out of control. If they don't panic, that helps their lungs to fill up."

The next doctor talked about a yogic procedure he learned at a seminar in California and later incorporated into his practice: "It started about ten years ago when a friend asked if I would be interested in going to a weekend meditation retreat. I was introduced to asana meditation and was so impressed by what happened that it became a regular part of my life. First of all, I became more self-aware and saw how out of focus my life was. It was a humiliation, but I was then able to make some necessary changes and improve my life. I began to use some of the methods in my practice, not necessarily meditation but teaching patients a way to observe their emotions and thoughts and to engage negative experiences instead of pushing away from them, which is what most people do.

"For example, when you're in the asana meditation, it focuses on body sensations. If the body sensation happens to be an itch or a pain or an ache, instead of changing your position or putting it out of your mind, you go right into the sensation of pain. When you do that, rather than the pain getting worse, it will actually resolve. I found that very useful. I use it to treat physical as well as psychological pain.

"I noticed that when patients talk about their emotional pain their bodies tended to become rather tense and their breathing retarded. I could hardly see their chests moving. So I had them pay attention to their body processes. When something happens that's painful, instead of tensing the muscles and holding the breath, which is how most people control their emotions, I teach them to notice where the tension is and to breathe into those places.

"I also use yogic breathing for headaches and chronic pain. As a result, patients use less pain medication. I have them do it as soon as they feel pain, instead of automatically grabbing for a pill. It helps bring the pain under their control. I might have them close their eyes and just breathe normally, to exhale and to focus their attention on the area of their body that's in pain. I might have them describe it: what the shape of it is and how deep it goes, or what color it is. You use all the senses. If you attend to your pain, it starts to dissolve."

THE AYURVEDIC SYSTEM

Perhaps the oldest medical system in the world (by some accounts it is 5,000 years old), India's Ayurveda is principally oriented toward prevention. It aims at achieving a state of physiological balance through a variety of natural procedures, including plant-based remedies, purification rituals, and familiar forms of yoga and meditation. We met a number of physicians who have picked up a remedy or two from the Ayurvedic tradition, but two of them have actually received special training in the system. One has incorporated it into a traditional Western practice; the other has devoted himself almost full-time to Ayurvedic practices. The first is an Orange County cardiologist:

"In 1971 I was going through the stress of medical school. I was getting very tired, and I needed something to relax me. My parents thought I was too sedentary, so they gave me a year's membership to a YMCA. The first week I went to the Y there was a lecture on Transcendental Meditation. I started doing it, and I found that I didn't burn out the way other students did. As the years went on, I was still able to retain a lot of vigor and enthusiasm.

"Some colleagues and I did research on patients with angina pectoris. We compiled data on one group while they exercised, and had another group do meditation on a regular basis. When both groups returned after six months, we again monitored them while they exercised. It turned out that the meditating group could exercise longer without pain than the control group. Their heart rate and blood pressure did not rise as quickly. So I started recommending TM to those patients who seemed receptive."

His interest in meditation eventually led him to investigate Ayurvedic medicine: "Around 1988 my patients started saying, 'Doctor, why don't you get into prevention? I don't want to take any more drugs.' I kept hearing that constant refrain, so finally I decided to look into it. At the time, Ayurveda was being promoted by the TM organization, the product of many years of development by Ayurvedic specialists and Maharishi Mahesh Yogi. Ayurveda appealed to me because it's natural and cost-effective. Before, I would recommend exercise, diet, and meditation for prevention. Now, I've added Ayurveda to my repertoire."

Like most of our interviewees, he insisted that he remains faithful to his formal training. "Western medicine is essential for people who are acutely ill and need a quick fix. That's the bulk of my patients. But once the emergency is over, prevention becomes the primary issue, and for that I've found nothing better than Ayurveda. It has helped me with a lot of difficult situations. For example, someone who is recuperating from a heart attack is usually given medication to thin the blood and dilate the arteries. I had a patient who could not tolerate any medicine. It upset his stomach, affected his liver, or caused other side effects. I gave him an Ayurvedic herbal preparation called Amrit Kalash, which has been shown to help the body process cholesterol and thin the blood. It's an ancient formula made of several exotic herbs, and it proved most helpful for that patient without any side effects."

The cardiologist said that he also prescribed Ayurvedic purification procedures: "The patients go to one of the Ayurvedic clinics and get an intensive treatment for a week or two. The body is essentially purified of toxins and impurities in a natural, but very profound way."

One of the doctor's star patients was a woman who came to him with a heart condition called mitral valve prolapse. "She had advanced breast cancer. Both breasts had been removed, and the malignancy had spread to her bones while she was pregnant. She was told it was hopeless and that in the past twenty years they had seen only one patient survive six months with her condition. Essentially, they gave her a death sentence. I was seeing her for her heart, which was almost incidental—a nuisance condition. But she asked me what could be done about the cancer. I didn't feel qualified to do anything, so I sent her to an Ayurvedic clinic in Massachusetts, where they gave her an intensive program of purification, extensive meditation, and special herbs. She went there three times and had remarkable experiences. During some of the techniques, she said she could feel something going on in her bones, like corn popping. In any event, the cancer is gone. Oncologists scratch their heads and say, 'I'm happy for her.' They can't explain it. We check her periodically, and everything seems fine. Her bone scans appear normal."

He also uses procedures from the Ayurvedic tradition of aroma-therapy. "Aromatherapy is a way of diffusing certain aromatic essential oils into the air. There are a number of blends, which we use for different purposes. My son has asthma. When it acts up, if it's a mild case, I can use aromatherapy and herbal tea to break up the attack. If it doesn't work, I use Western approaches—inhalers and broncho-dilaters."

The other Ayurvedic advocate we met was a family practitioner who had previously been unimpressed by alternative medicine: "I had an open attitude, but I couldn't embrace those practices in the absence of good, rigorous research. Ayurveda has been around so long— thousands of years of empirical experience—so I felt it was more valid." He now runs an Ayurvedic clinic in the Los Angeles area.

He explained a fundamental precept of Ayurveda: "It revolves around the concept of *doshas,* three metabolic principles that govern individual physiology: *vatta,* which is responsible for all movement in the body; *pitta,* which produces energy and heat, and governs digestion; and *kapha,* which provides the body's substance and solidity. The relative proportion of these three forces determines a person's body type. The first thing an Ayurvedic physician does is determine the patient's body type, which in turn influences the treatment plan for any given diagnosis.

"With every patient I use a pulse diagnosis and a questionnaire to determine his constitutional type. This, along with the specific symptoms, determines the course of treatment. Imbalances of the three *doshas* can be discerned in the pulse by the volume, viscosity, undulations on the arterial wall, and other subtle changes that can be picked up with training. Based on these factors, we recommend a treatment plan."

The treatments in his repertoire include meditation, yogic exercises, purification procedures, and recommendations for dietary and behavioral changes. With respect to that last element, he said, "It has to do with conducting life in tune with the rhythms of nature. For example, in Ayurveda, hypertension can result from different imbalances—too much *vatta* or *pitta*. We go after the predominant *dosha*. Some patients still require medication, but I rarely just prescribe drugs the first time I see them, unless their blood pressure is sky-high. Most people don't have a critical level, so I use a multipronged approach— diet, meditation, exercises, and the like for four to six months. For example, with a hard-driving man with a lot of frustration, time pressure, and hostility, I recommended cooling foods as opposed to hot, spicy foods or pungent, salty foods. Plus, I prescribe herbal preparations for pacifying *pitta*.

"We also work with thought and attitude. I believe that the thoughts we have actually structure the molecules in the brain, and every time we change the brain chemistry, it affects our mood, outlook, behavior, and physical senses. It's just as real as getting a vein full of Valium. It's not just a matter of positive thinking. The problem with positive thinking is that people feel guilty if they have negative thoughts. I advocate simplicity and effortlessness. If you feel you have the choice of favoring something positive, then you can do it. You don't have to ignore a problem to have a positive attitude about it."

HOMEOPATHY

The other system that appealed to a number of physicians in our sample is actually enjoying a resurgence. Homeopathy originated in the eighteenth century with the work of German physician Samuel Hahnemann. By the early part of this century, it boasted a considerable following in America. As many as a quarter of all physicians were trained in homeopathic medical schools; one hundred hospitals used the system and homeopathic pharmacies were common. But homeopathy was a victim of the social and political upheaval that transformed medicine in the U.S. While it retained its legitimacy in Europe, it was not until the 1960s that interest in the system was revived in America.

The first two excerpts are from doctors who have switched almost entirely to homeopathic medicine. The first has a family practice in the San Fernando Valley: "I came out of medical school very idealistic. But, after being in private practice and working in hospitals for three years, it became apparent that there were distinct flaws in what I'd been taught. Too many patients weren't getting better. If I cured one cold, they'd have five or six more. People who lost weight would gain it back. People who were depressed were still depressed. So I embarked on a self-study program to examine alternatives. I studied everything from herbal medicine to nutrition and from acupuncture to iridology—the whole gamut. I felt there must be something more I could do. I wasn't throwing out my training, I just wanted to supplement it with other methods."

The pivotal event occurred when the doctor was suddenly cast in the role of patient: "I was at a friend's house, and I hit my knee—banged the patella on a coffee table. Immediately, a bruise started to appear. It swelled up and was very painful. My friend ran up to me saying, 'Oh, take this, take this.' I looked down and saw these tiny, itty-bitty tablets. I thought, 'Well, I'll humor her. They're so small, they can't possibly affect me.'

"So I took them, and a few hours later, when I was changing for bed, that big bruise was gone. I couldn't remember which knee I'd hit. I poked it—no pain. Nothing. I thought, 'This couldn't happen! Bruises like that take two weeks to heal.' Usually you can't poke such a bruise. So, I had a choice: I could either ignore what I'd seen because I couldn't explain it, or I could find out more, which meant my belief system was going to have to be stretched. I had an intuitive feeling that if I started looking into this, my life was going to be turned upside down. But it was too dramatic to ignore. I read some books on homeopathy, and at one point, I thought, 'This is what I've been looking for.' It's like when you fall in love—that moment of recognition: here it is."

After extensive studies in the U.S. and Europe, she started a homeopathic practice separate from her regular practice. She explained the fundamental premises of the system: "Fundamentally, homeopathy states that everything that happens to us, everything we think and feel, everything that's physically wrong with us, is connected. To a homeopath, a symptom means any characteristic from any aspect of the person. Therefore, symptoms include all the complaints from the body, as well as emotions, thoughts, reactions to stress or weather conditions, sleep patterns, food preferences, family, social and work experiences, and other areas. In cases of chronic illness it can take up to two hours to collect enough information before the proper prescription can be made. This individualization is a key feature of homeopathy.

"There are over two thousand homeopathic remedies that are derived from plants and minerals, or from a few animal substances. Their principle is fundamentally opposite that of allopathic medicine's where symptoms represent a malfunction and have to be suppressed. In homeopathy, symptoms are created by the body during its process of protecting itself. The remedies naturally activate the body's own ability for self-healing. They help eliminate the reason the body developed the symptoms in the first place. Prescribing is based on a biological principle called the Law of Similars, which states that when you give a healthy person a particular substance, certain distinct symptoms will appear. If you see that constellation of symptoms in a sick person, then that same substance will cure him. A homeopathic remedy gives the body a little more of what it needs to fight the disease."

Homeopaths claim that their remedies are created by a unique processing method that retains the healing power of the original substance while removing its potential side effects. No one knows exactly how the remedies work, and no conclusive studies have confirmed their effectiveness. "Homeopathy in this day and age is an empirical system," said our source. "Our opponents hold that against us, but the history of medicine is replete with remedies that are empirically useful for years before there was an adequate scientific explanation."

The doctor offered to describe her favorite cases: "Often people come in for something very different than their fundamental pathology. One was a prominent executive of a Fortune 500 company. She was getting frequent colds and had chronic headaches. She was taking about two bottles of aspirin a week. However, she also had a severe, lifelong depression. She never really wanted to go into the field she was in, but because of various pressures—family, peers, and so on—she'd done it and had excelled. But still she had this internal feeling of hopelessness. She was pretty startled that the interview turned to her depression because it was not what she came in for. The upshot was that I gave her a remedy, and within a month, she had no more headaches and her energy increased. Within a year she quit her job and started doing some art work, something she'd always wanted to do. Now she's a very successful artist, and she's very happy. The remedy I used was aurum—homeopathic gold. The character of aurum is somebody who is very striving, who has to be the best, but also has an internal sense of worthlessness—'I'm unworthy.' That's where her depression came from. I use aurum a lot with suicidal patients and children whose parents pressure them to achieve."

She was eager to speak of a multiple sclerosis patient: "She's a thirty-two-year-old woman who had her first sign of MS at the age of fourteen, but wasn't diagnosed until she was twenty-nine years old. She'd had joint pains and visual problems all along. Then she developed numbness, tingling, and weakness in the leg, and suddenly half of her body went numb, and they informed her she had MS. Basically, MS is a downhill course. It's not a pretty picture. So she came to me, and I gave her hemlock canian. There are about thirty remedies that we use for MS, but this is one of the major ones.

"In about a month she was doing something most patients do when they start getting better—they don't quite believe it. She didn't want to be too enthusiastic, just in case it was a fluke. But her eye symptoms completely went away. The strength in her legs improved. She could walk up and down stairs. Her energy increased. Her mind was clearer. She could make it all day without taking a nap. Before, she couldn't stoop down and stand up. Now she could. Her walking and visual symptoms improved. All the fuzziness and dullness was gone. It's been about six months now, and her joint pain is completely gone."

Remarkable MS remissions often occur but usually are not lasting, so it leaves the ultimate certainty of this treatment tantalizing but yet unproven.

Despite her convictions about homeopathy, the doctor still uses mainstream treatments and diagnostic procedures: "I had a patient who had all the symptoms of gallstones. I thought, I'd better check that out. I took an ultra-sound, and her gallstones were the size of gooseberries, so I recommended surgery. Now, if she had come to me earlier, she might never have had a gallstone. But by the time they were that big, she needed surgery."

Another doctor began his career as a cardiologist only to turn exclusively to homeopathy several years later. He told us how that transformation came about: "I had hurt my leg by running forty miles a week. I tried everything to heal it, but nothing worked. I had heard about homeopathy, but I never paid much attention to it. Then one day, while my knee was aching, I said, well, I'll give it a try. So I went to the homeopathic drug store, and I looked in the little book and found a remedy that seemed to fit. I took a dose, and my knee improved a little. It wasn't dramatic, but I *felt* wonderful. I got this marvelous burst of energy. So I said to myself, 'I'm going to study this.'

"I studied on my own and signed up for some seminars, but I didn't treat anyone for another year. I had a patient who had recurring urinary tract infections. I put her on antibiotics, and ten days into the treatment she relapsed. So I said to her, 'I've been studying this stuff. If you'd like to try it, I'll see if I can find a remedy.' She said she'd try anything. So I gave her a remedy—lycopodium clavatis—and it was the most dramatic thing I'd ever seen. Not only did it eradicate the urinary tract infection, which I confirmed with a urine culture, but it changed her whole life."

He subsequently turned to homeopathy full-time. He told us of successful cures for premenstrual syndrome, broken bones, bee stings, ear infections, and other ailments. Here are just two: "I have a patient who was on allopathic medicine for ulcerative colitis. He had some response to it, but he had to take the medicine four times a day and he still had the colitis. Interestingly, in taking his history, I found that he was eating huge amounts of jalapeño peppers and spicy food, which I knew might be rough on his colon. I had him eliminate spicy foods, and there was a fifty percent improvement in his condition. His gastroenterologist never even thought to ask him what he ate. Then I gave him a remedy that helped him a bit, but it wasn't quite right. Then I tried homeopathic sulphur, and the ulcerative colitis cleared up. We stopped the other medication and repeated the homeopathic remedy two or three times. He's now gone six weeks without any problems."

He told the next story to emphasize the art of finding the right remedy: "The patient was bedridden with a bad back and terrible sciatica. An internist had him on muscle relaxants and thought he might need surgery for a herniated disc. I gave him a particular remedy. The next day, no go. I gave it to him again, only a stronger dose. No change. I gave him a different remedy. Nothing. He was still bedridden. The only position he was comfortable in was lying down. So I found a description of a form of sciatica that felt better lying down, worse sitting, and intermediate standing up. I gave him a pill for that specific syndrome and told him to take another one at bedtime. The next morning at eight A.M., the phone rang, and he said, 'That stuff really works!' I gave him another dose two or three days later, and he was completely well. But the two previous remedies hadn't done anything. That's why it's so hard to study homeopathy in a controlled, scientific way."

Several doctors who dabble in homeopathy advocated the use of the remedy arnica for traumas such as bruises or sprains. One general practitioner near San Diego told us a dramatic story, in which arnica was used for a psychological trauma: "A woman about forty years old came to me with a history of choking sensations during sleep. Every night, after about an hour of sleep, she woke up choking. She would get up and walk around, then go back to sleep for an hour, then get up again. She was always tired. She'd been to doctors everywhere. They gave her tranquilizers and antidepressants, and nothing did any good.

"She came to me, and I tried this, I tried that, and then I thought, maybe there are remedies in homeopathy that can help. So I questioned her, and at one point I asked if she'd had any emotional traumas as a child. She said that if she did something wrong around the house—dirtied or broke something—her father used to wake her up, grab her by the neck, and spank her. She couldn't go back to sleep for fear that he would come back and beat her again.

"So I connected that to her presenting complaint: 'Subconsciously, you think your father is going to come in and spank you.' She said, 'I know that, but it doesn't help me with my problem.' So, I thought, maybe arnica would apply to a mental trauma as well as a physical one. I gave it to her and didn't see her for two or three weeks. When she came back, she said she'd been sleeping well for the first time in twenty years. It surprised me. It was a very unusual recovery from something that had lasted so long."

A Santa Monica physician who includes homeopathy in a remarkably varied repertoire told us these stories: "I went to a patient's house. She was very sick with diarrhea and vomiting, and she thought she had food poisoning. I looked at her and said, 'You're the picture of arsenic poisoning.' So I gave her some homeopathic arsenic. She was supposed to play tennis that day and had been lying on the couch moaning. But after I treated her, she got into the elevator and said, 'I'm well,' and went to play three sets of tennis.

"Then there was a thirty-eight-year-old woman who came to see me after receiving the usual treatment for measles. Her quality of life and her vitality were not fully restored. She had lost her sense of smell, had hair loss, and was fatigued. She had wanted to get pregnant again, but felt she was too weak. So I gave her posatela and homeopathic measles. She came back two weeks later and said, 'It's a miracle.' Her hair stopped falling out, her sense of smell was starting to come back, and she felt great. Now she was talking about getting pregnant again. I wish I could say every patient had that experience."

The same doctor told us about an intriguing variation of homeopathy: "To me, every patient's prescription is sort of my art work. It's like an improvisation. For instance, I might take homeopathic Epstein-Barr virus and inject it into a kidney point on a specific acupuncture circuit. Injecting homeopathic compounds is a common practice in Germany. Let's say somebody's fatigued. I'll take homeopathic Vitamin B-12 and inject it into an acupuncture point, and they'll get much more energy from that than if I'd done it in the arm or the buttocks."

Our final excerpts are from a general practitioner who, while practicing in Europe, came across an extraordinary treatment modality from traditional Tibetan medicine that incorporated principles of acupuncture and homeopathy: "I've gotten many remedies by reading about ancient styles of practices. I read in a Tibetan text about homeopathic preparations of blood drawn from areas associated with a particular disease. I used it a few times. You extract two or three drops of blood from a vein that crosses an acupuncture point that corresponds with the patient's condition. Then you prepare a liquid homeopathic solution. You gradually dilute it and use a process called secussion, which is basically hitting the vial that the liquid is in. You take an extract of something and secuss it into a solution. In this case, the extract was blood. The patient takes it orally. It's his own blood; there's no transfer to or from another person."

He said he used this curious treatment on a few patients who did not respond to ordinary remedies: "There was a patient with Raynaud's phenomenon—an uncontrollable constriction and flushing of the distal extremities. The fingers and toes get cold and white, then very red. It's painful, and sometimes it becomes gangrenous. The standard drugs sometimes work, but patients don't like the side effects. And in this case, the patient had already tried the medications.

"I drew blood from a point on the 'triple warmer' meridian, near the tip of the finger. I had the patient take three drops of the diluted blood solution under the tongue, three times a day. It went on for three or four weeks. Solutions in homeopathy are so diluted that a few drops of blood go a very long way. It helped quite a lot. I have to admit, I can't explain it in scientific terms. Theoretically, every part of the body has its own physiology, so the blood might reflect some subtle local properties. I know that sounds strange, but there might be something that reflects whatever the disorder is. According to homeopathic theory, that property can be used to correct it."

The physician said he also used this form of treatment on several women with dysmenorrhea. "In my experience, dysfunctions with no specific physiological abnormalities are most responsive to these 'natural' treatments. Dysmenorrhea is a classic. Women have pain around the time of their menses, and we can't always explain why. All you can do is use pain killers or minerals to reduce the force of contraction of the uterine wall. But basically the pain is always there. I had found acupuncture effective, but when I used the Tibetan blood treatment, it was even better. I used points on the abdomen, along the conception vessel meridian. They would take the treatment, and the next time they got their period it wasn't as severe as before. Some of the patients got completely better."

One has to ask why doctors are interested in systems of medicine that could easily be dismissed as antiquated or even primitive. I believe it indicates a respect for medical traditions other than our own, and a pragmatism that compels us to look for new ideas and procedures that might enhance our therapeutic capabilities and generate new hypotheses. It seems likely that over time, effective elements of systems other than our own will be further adapted to contemporary needs. As in the arts, medical science can only benefit from judicious cross-fertilization.

CHAPTER 8

THE SPIRIT OF HEALING

"R eligious medicine is timeless," wrote Henry E. Sigerist in his definitive book, *A History of Medicine:* "We come upon it in the initial stages and throughout the course of every civilization, no matter what other forms of medicine may have been developed."

In virtually every culture, there are, and have always been, afflicted individuals who turn to magico-religious practitioners for help. Shamans, sorcerers, and priests who view themselves as agents of the divine or custodians of magical powers have always existed side by side with healers whose work is based on rational-empirical principles. Even in ancient Greece, where Hippocrates founded the tradition of Western empirical medicine, there existed a simultaneous belief that deities intervened in the healing process. At Epidaurus, often considered the precursor of the modern hospital, there were invocations to the gods, and at its center was a temple devoted to Aesculapius, a quasi-deity whom Zeus had named the god of medicine. "The Epidaurian pattern of the cult of Aesculapius," writes Sigerist, "was followed in other Greek and Roman sanctuaries, and its ritual was even continued in Christian churches."

This belief in the healing power of non-physical forces both within and without the individual has never disappeared, even though it has not been countenanced by medical science. This is evidenced in the linguistic root of the word 'heal'; it stems from the German 'hailaz' and the Old English 'hal,' roots that are shared by the modern words 'holy' and 'whole.' It remains an article of faith in many religious groups and a private conviction of countless patients and physicians (about forty years ago, for example, the number of Christian Science practitioners in America rivaled that of M.D.s). When holistic physicians added spiritual aspects to those qualities of human life that are known to affect health, the metaphysics of healing took on a modern, nonsectarian visage, divorced from organized religion.

In this chapter, we will be examining the spiritual side of the ancient dichotomy between magico-religious and rational-empirical approaches to medicine. From our interviews, it would appear that some physicians are metaphysicians as well. A surprising number of our doctors chose to speak of matters that can only be called spiritual. In some cases, their remarks centered on the medical value of faith, whether in the conventional, religious sense, or as it relates to some nameless higher power, or in the Star Wars sense of an inner, empowering Force. A number of physicians attested to a belief in Eastern philosophy or in a private cosmology influenced by mysticism and modern physics. In some cases, their beliefs took pragmatic form in practices such as meditation, psychic powers, or prayer. We begin with some broad statements from physicians about the spiritual dimension of their work.

First, a family doctor and professor at an East Coast medical school: "I've always had a sense of something beyond the mechanistic and the behavioral. It's a hierarchy of knowing. The biological sciences are absolutely necessary for understanding how we work on the physical level. But unfortunately, not all physicians make use of the healing elements inherent in one's emotional and interpersonal life. In the same way, those who don't understand the spiritual dimension in human functioning miss another, perhaps even more powerful, influence. There was an evolution in my understanding of the behavioral vectors of illness, and it took a few more years to appreciate that the best psychologists and psychiatrists can't adequately explain the nature of the disease process without some consideration of the spiritual malaise involved."

A Los Angeles physician who encourages patients to do yoga, meditation, Tai Chi, or float in the hermetically sealed salt-water tank in his office, told us: "In medical school we're taught that illnesses are pathology. In terms of my spiritual understanding, diseases may also create a crisis in consciousness, or in the Chinese sense, a dangerous opportunity."

For the following general practitioner, the term "spiritual" has a specific medical orientation: "Healing people and understanding illness involve something far greater than the training I've received. Sometimes it seems that there's a basic imperfection in the fact that people take care of other people, since we're all so vulnerable and prone to errors ourselves. Yet, I feel there's something very spiritual about the interaction between doctor and patient. I'm only beginning to understand that connection.

"I see people who have the will and determination to overcome their illnesses and live. By and large, I think people do a lot on their own, and probably the best care one can give patients is to restore their energy and encourage a sense of personal responsibility for their well-being."

THE ROAD TO DAMASCUS

Several physicians told us that personal epiphanies and spiritual quests have had a strong influence on their practices, altering the way they view their patients and, in some cases, opening the way to uncommon healing techniques as well. One was an osteopathic physician, who had a mystical experience when he was twelve:

"It was an ecstatic feeling of a great light entering my body, which nobody could explain to me. My mother thought that I was possessed by the devil. It had a major impact on my life, and I began a lifelong study of transcendental phenomena."

We asked how those formative studies influenced his subsequent training and practice as a physician: "I think it helped me understand that as physicians we can simply act as catalysts for the expression of that healing spirit within us. I believed that the liberation of one's spiritual forces can optimize healing, and I looked for methods that would not countermand the wisdom of the body by suppressing it with allopathic drugs or surgery. However, I understand their necessity in the care of traumas and growths that require surgery, or diseases that are drug-specific. But I treat the patient without disturbing the homeostatic process. Taoist philosophy taught me at an early age that whatever you do to the body has an impact on its spirit, mind, and emotions.

"My belief in my Creator is very important in my work. I see medicine as a calling. That's one of the reasons I do my spiritual practices every morning. I have a series of exercises—Taoist yogic techniques—which allow me to open up and relate to my patients in as loving a way as I possibly can."

He said that he sometimes teaches his patients the techniques he himself practices: "Especially with patients who have a spiritual leaning, I'll often teach meditative techniques—for instance, the so-called microcosmic orbit. It involves a meditation in which energy is drawn down through the pineal body—third-eye area—into the tongue and on down through the central part of the body to the perineum—the area between the sexual organs and the anus. It entails repetitions of drawing the energy up the spine on inhalation and down the body on exhalation." He indicated that those patients who practice this find it most beneficial for relaxation.

A Los Angeles practitioner told us that he believes in the healing value of ritual and sometimes composes special ceremonies for his patients: "A woman came in with severe, incapacitating migraine headaches. She had been divorced for ten years and was remarried, but she never divorced emotionally. Her first husband was a physician, and she was still clinging to her former identity as his wife. I believed that the previous marriage ritual predominated and the divorce ritual was relatively ineffective or so painful she blocked it out. She hadn't really released the first marriage, and I felt that the migraines were the result of an emotional impasse.

"We created a divorce ceremony. We asked her to write about how she viewed her identity then and who she now believed herself to be. We then held a burning ritual; she had to burn a picture of herself with her first husband while she read the new affirmation of herself. This was six months ago, and, to my knowledge, she has not had any migraine headaches since."

The next two respondents are psychiatrists whose ideas were transformed by their exploration of what one termed the transpersonal view. "As I pursued my own spiritual growth, I would bring my experience into my work insofar as my patients could accept it. Sometimes I suggest that people meditate, or I meditate with them. It's a form of non-verbal communication that enhances rapport."

She told us of a program called the Spiritual Emergency Network: "People having spiritual breakthroughs can sometimes seem psychotic. They may be going through a spiritual crisis and often have the conviction that they're in contact with God. This can be misinterpreted as paranoid schizophrenia or a manic episode, and they are usually put on antipsychotic drugs that abort the process. Psychiatric hospitals are the worst possible places for these people, who are in an extremely open and sensitive state. Those undergoing a spiritual crisis must be in a safe, positive healing environment and among supportive people who are aware of the transformation they're undergoing and can help them reach a higher level of integration."

The psychiatrist told us of a young man who was referred to her because he was hearing voices. "He was withdrawn and frightened and appeared psychotic. This happened after an insightful psychedelic experience, which released a lot of emotional and spiritual material. It resolved after two psychotherapy sessions. I don't believe it was a typical psychotic break. There was no suggestive history."

She believes that the outcome would not have been as positive had the young man been treated by someone who did not understand spiritual emergencies: "He might have been diagnosed schizophrenic and treated inappropriately. It was a breakthrough, not a breakdown."

The next psychiatrist said that her studies of mysticism, ritual, and non-Western philosophies have helped her to treat patients more effectively. "What I do now is like a soul therapy. Before doing all this personal work, I wasn't really in touch with different planes of consciousness and had no concept of what the soul was. Now I have a sense of the essence of people. If one can get in touch with that, he will get well."

In describing her work with schizophrenics, her conversation became rather esoteric: "I have a deeper understanding of the schizophrenic process than I ever had before. I recognize schizophrenics as being caught on some other planes of consciousness. They can't differentiate between fantasy and reality; physical space and time have a different meaning. I believe that I can make contact with them and see where they're coming from. I try to get in touch with that part of them that can tell where they are."

We asked what she meant by "making contact": "In my mind and in my spirit. I enter their delusions and attempt a kind of confrontation to try to help them get in touch with reality. It's as if they have to learn again what reality is. It does take time."

We asked if she eschews conventional treatment, such as psychoactive medication. "No, I use drugs if the patients are suicidal or manic and I don't have the luxury of doing this kind of intervention. It's very difficult, and I don't have the energy to work with many people that way. But when I do, it's remarkable. For example, this one girl was a beautiful model around eighteen or nineteen. She had taken cocaine and found herself in a mental hospital and didn't know why. Her family told me she had become wild and incoherent and was extremely suspicious and abusive toward her mother.

"It became apparent that the mother was intent upon her daughter becoming a movie star. She was extremely possessive. At times, my patient feared that her mother was trying to rape and kill her. She's an intelligent woman and very creative. Sometimes she'll have visions of God and angels and describe heavenly scenes. I'm trying to show her how to transform her creative imagination into some form of artistic expression.

"I think the psychiatry that we learn in medical school and in residency would just say this is a psychotic delusion and we should get her out of it as fast as possible with large doses of drugs. But if I can convert hate-filled delusions, like the ones about her mother, to spiritual ones, then it could lead her to a higher dimension."

As our interview progressed, the psychiatrist discussed her views about two perplexing areas of human existence, sex and death: "I've cured several patients of impotency and frigidity with transformational work and chanting. I've used it mostly with men, and a few women. I created a chant that essentially activates the sexual center. This takes place after the preliminary workup, which involves a detailed sexual history and physical examination. I check for any contributing diseases, especially diabetes, alcohol abuse, or atherosclerosis."

She then told us how her spiritual journey has affected the way she works with the dying: "I try to help people see the dying process as a transition and as a movement of their soul. When I feel that a patient is really entering the dying process, I don't treat it like mourning or sadness, but like a festival and a celebration, an opening up to an extraordinary adventure. I believe that there is no death as we know it. We develop into a larger consciousness that isn't grounded in a physical body, but moves into spirit until it fuses with the divine. I'm not exactly sure where it goes, but I do believe that other levels exist. They're not places but states of consciousness, and it's important that people who are with the dying don't try to hold them back from going on to the expanded consciousness they need to reach.

"I try to help the dying to make the passage consciously, so they understand it's not the end, and they die without agitation, pain, or the need to be sedated. It is my belief that they die in a state of love and peacefulness, knowing that they are going to go on to a greater enlightenment.

"I was asked to see a man and his wife. She had been dying for months, just hanging on the edge. She'd had breast cancer, and it had spread all over her body. I told her husband, 'Your wife has already gone. There is just this body left; she's staying here because you don't want to let her go. You have to release her.' Soon after his wife died, he called to thank me and said, 'I really miss her, but I know that I was holding her back.' "

We asked the doctor how she would deal with a dying patient who did not share her views of the afterlife: "I talk to them openly and tell them that it's very important, before you make this passage, to clean up any unfinished business. If you have anything to say to your children, or if you're holding anything back, this is the time to address those issues. Holding fear, resentment, guilt, or any kind of negative feeling will make it more difficult for you. So I tell them to empty themselves. For example, the woman with breast cancer called her daughter, and they spent a couple of hours making peace with one another. It was a very big release for her, and it was most significant for the daughter, too. Your readers are going to think I'm nuts, but I believe that it's imperative to work in this fashion and for the family to be there and be supportive."

THE HEALING POWER OF PRAYER

A Pennsylvania physician told us that the only unconventional aspect of his practice is that he prays for, and sometimes with, his patients: "A large percentage of my patients share a belief structure that allows them to benefit from prayer. Among the questions I've learned to ask is, 'When you are under the greatest stress or have the most concerns, where do you turn for support and counsel?' This is a very revealing question. It gives the doctor an ally. Patients may say they turn to family and friends, or they turn inward, or they read the great masters, or might say, 'I don't have anyone.' But often, I am told, 'I go to the Lord in prayer.' It's remarkable how frequently I hear that.

"I regard prayer as a source of organized help, like family and friends. I remind them that they can use whatever's worked in the past. I encourage them to share it with clergy if that's where their strength lies, or to use whatever scriptures they believe. Occasionally, I might suggest that we pray together concerning their condition. But, I don't do that unless I've established a long-term relationship."

He remembered an elderly patient with trigeminal neuralgia, also known as tic douloureux: "It's characterized by excruciating pain in the face that is incapacitating. If it recurs over a long period, the patient can become very depressed, even to the point of suicide. This was the case with this gentlemen. He'd been to a number of specialists, and was now considering neurosurgery.

"When I saw how his emotional situation was deteriorating, I volunteered that we should pray about it. We did, and he broke down and tearfully said that he had never shared a prayer with a physician before. Over the weeks and months after that, he said the pain was gradually going away. We stopped talking about neurosurgery and decreased the medication to almost nothing. The condition remained in a low-grade fashion. He would occasionally feel it, but it was never again the terrible pain that was bringing him despair."

We asked how he, as a physician, could explain the effect of prayer: "I believe it was divine intervention and that he was able to make use of his conviction that such a power exists. I mean, he believed that God was hearing his prayer and easing his pain."

He said that he prays in solitude daily, sometimes for specific patients, but usually to entreat God to make him a better physician: "I pray that I might be sensitive to my patients' problems, that I become aware of hidden agendas that people bring, and that I might use my skills most appropriately."

A family practitioner in Northern California described a personal transformation that led him to incorporate prayer into his medical practice on occasion.: "I've seen some incredible things that didn't make any sense at all. One was the case of an old woman who died suddenly in a grocery store. When she got to the emergency room, attempts to save her failed. She was clearly brain dead, so I just turned her over to the interns and went to bed.

"The next morning I got a call from the doctors, and they said they couldn't believe it, but the patient was showing signs of alertness. I said, 'Don't kid yourselves, there's no way.' They said, 'Oh, yeah, she's trying to pull the tubes out.' So I go up there, and she's wide awake, gesticulating with this thing in her throat. There's just no reason that she should have been alive. It was a miracle."

That and other extraordinary instances of recovery, he said, made him accept the unpredictable and mysterious aspects of medicine and rethink his philosophy of life: "It was a funny thing. I didn't have real strong religious beliefs when I started my training program. Now, I really believe that there's a spiritual side of life that we're not aware of, either by choice or by blindness. You can see that these chairs are solid, and you know there are walls we can't pass through, but if there's anything to atomic theory, they're actually seething masses of electrons. There are two realities: a reality I can sit on and lean against and a reality that can be turned into energy. I think the same is true of us. I think we have a spiritual reality that we're not aware of, and I think that, for some reason, God didn't want that woman to die at that time."

He said that his spiritual beliefs changed the way he views the physician's role: "Only the most self-glorified person would think he's doing the actual healing. Getting well is *facilitated* by medicine, but healing involves more than doctoring. That's why I try to minimize medication in favor of education and lifestyle changes."

It is also why he has, on occasion, resorted to prayer: "Once, when I was on duty in the hospital, we got this phone call from a minister's wife. She was in absolute anguish. She and her husband were on vacation up in the Sierras. She was pregnant, and they had two small children in the car, and the car stalled. The husband was pushing the car up a hill and suddenly fell to the ground, and he couldn't move because of an excruciating pain in the back of his neck. It was obviously a hemorrhage.

"The agony in that woman's voice was awful. I didn't know what to do. I was sitting there with people all around me as I talked on the phone, and I just felt like I needed to pray. She and I started praying over the telephone, and I suddenly felt this assurance that everything was going to be okay. And, as the husband began to come around, the prayers started changing to thanksgivings. I was just thankful that he was being spared. I also noticed how quiet it was in the room because everybody was shocked at this hard-nosed doctor who was suddenly praying.

"I believe there is a God who is sovereign, who will let us be a part of the divine plan or not, depending on our choice. It's his will that he can heal somebody whether I pray or not."

An ear, nose, and throat specialist in Los Angeles told us this story: "A young lady, whom I had known since her teens, was brought to me in a wheelchair one day. She was about twenty-two at the time and had contracted multiple sclerosis. She determinedly told me, 'I'm going to get well. I've organized a prayer group among my friends. Someone is always praying for me, around the clock.' There were about two dozen people whom she knew through some organization. I don't think it was church-oriented.

"Well, about six months later, she came in on her own two feet. She said, 'I'm perfectly well.' I let her squeeze my hand. I checked her reflexes. There was nothing left of the MS. Nothing. I've seen her once more, maybe two or three years after that, and she was still doing well." Spontaneous remission is known to occur with MS patients, the doctor acknowledged, but he believed that this case was not a typical remission.

Some of our prayerful physicians use unconventional methods as opposed to the usual prayers of supplication. One internist devotes time in his personal meditations to his patients: "I visualize them as healthy or doing something with me sometime in the future. I don't believe in imagery where you say, 'Disease, go away.' I don't think that works. I think you have to visualize a person as being healthy. I do it quite often with people who are terminally ill. I also do it when I'm sick and for loved ones, whether they're my patients or not. I have a sister who has cancer, and I visualize her dancing at my son's wedding, about twenty-five years from now."

An internist told us how another spiritual group healed a patient with a form of prayer: "I'll give you an interesting story. This fellow developed a tumor at the base of the tongue. He had a biopsy and was told that it was malignant and would have to have what is called a radical neck section. They take out all the musculature and part of the base of the tongue as well. It's a disfiguring surgery, and people have difficulty speaking. Now, I have a rabbi friend whose work is oriented around mystical Judaism. He placed my patient on a table with about twenty people around it and had them focus their energy toward him. The next week, I called his surgeon and asked if we could put the surgery off for a month.

"The surgeon said, 'If we wait a month and go in there and find the tumor is even larger, would you be willing to accept that responsibility?' I said, 'It's up to the patient. But what if the tumor is benign?' The surgeon said, 'It's not benign. We have tissue diagnosis. It's malignant.' I said, 'What if it were to change to a benign tumor?' He said, 'Those things don't happen.' I told the patient all this. He elected to go ahead and have the surgery. Well, when they removed the tumor, it was totally benign."

THE ZEN OF HEALING

Several doctors spoke not of their own spiritual beliefs but of their patients'. Even physicians with determinedly secular attitudes felt that patients who draw strength or will power from religious faith might be in a more advantageous position than their nonbelieving counterparts. We even heard a number of remarkable healing stories that the doctors attributed to the power of spiritual conviction. First, a doctor who runs a clinic in Los Angeles explains why he often advises patients "to worship God and follow the precepts of their religious beliefs. I do it especially with patients with hypertension and other stress-related disorders. I think there is value to worship. There is a certain quality of surrender that comes about if they believe in divine intervention. It might also produce an inner transformation that has a salutary influence on destructive impulses like fear or self-pity, or generates more faith in getting better. For some people, it's something they've gotten away from, like having been an altar boy who felt good going to church, or loving the synagogue during holidays. For them, going back to their faith can be very nourishing."

Here is a story from a physician who specializes in industrial medicine: "I put this sixty-five-year-old patient in the hospital with severe abdominal pain. We did a barium enema and found some obstruction in the colon. We operated and he was full of cancer. He asked, 'How much time do I have?' I told him it looked like three or four months, and he said, 'No, you're talking about three or four *years.*' He was a deeply religious man. He had great faith that God wanted him to stay alive. He was very happy, very cheerful. In the hospital he would say, 'You're not going to kill me, and I'm going to prove it to you. I don't want to die, and I'm not going to sit down and brood about it.' He had radiation and chemotherapy, and it's now been six or seven years and he comes to me and says, 'You still want to bet?' His wife worries about him more than he does about himself. He says, 'Do something for my wife. She worries.' This was no ordinary remission. I'm convinced this man is alive today because of his faith."

The surgeon who told us the next story had the same conviction: "There's a lady I operated on who had twenty-three out of twenty-six lymph nodes positive for cancer. The primary cancer was at the base of the tongue. The chances of surviving for five years is something like zero to five percent. It's almost unheard of with as many lesions as she had in the neck. Any doctor would say she'd be dead in a year, or two at best. Never five. Well, she's been in remission for eighteen years. This woman had one of the strongest faiths I've ever seen. She belongs to a Protestant denomination and leads groups in her home for the terminally ill. She instills in them a tremendous amount of courage and fortitude to handle their own disease. I believe there is something there beyond what we know in medicine."

An emergency room physician in Palm Springs told us: "A spiritual outlook does seem to help. I remember one elderly lady who came in because she was constipated and also had some back pain. Well, we found that she had a pretty advanced case of cancer. When I told her, she seemed more concerned about her constipation than about this malignant disease. She understood the diagnosis, and she was well aware of the implications. I said, 'It doesn't seem to bother you very much,' and she then told me about something that happened twenty years earlier.

"She had been assaulted by a man, who hit her on the head and left her seemingly unconscious. She was aware of being outside her physical body and watching the assailant pound on her. Later, she had a similar experience when she had surgery to remove a blood clot and was again 'out of her body' watching the surgery. From her experiences, she felt certain that her physical body was really not all she was, so she could accept the fact that the cancer could possibly be lethal. She had a very good response to radiation treatment and was doing amazingly well when she moved away about a year later."

The doctor said he has encountered several patients like that woman. The power of their belief has influenced his attitude toward medicine: "It taught me how little I know and that I have to keep an open mind. I believe very strongly in the ability of people to face problems with some measure of joy and confidence. Enthusiasm greatly enhances the healing process. I wish that physicians were just as aware of the life of the spirit as they are of the body. I believe that many doctors are totally oblivious to any spiritual involvement and are completely divorced from the spiritual aspects of medicine."

Religious belief was also lauded by this orthopedic surgeon: "I've done a lot of spinal fusions for scoleosis, curvature of the spine. I find my religious patients always do better than those who are not. They fuse more rapidly than patients who don't believe. When I was a student, a surgeon told us about a young ballerina who developed a malignant tumor and was told that her leg would have to be amputated. She refused the surgery and she and her mother said they were just going to pray hard and hope for her recovery. She actually did get better without any treatment. This was confirmed by X-rays."

GNOSTIC DIAGNOSTICS

While medical technology has made the process of diagnosis more of a science than it once was, it still remains an art to a large extent. As with any art form, it entails a certain combination of reason and intuition. Most doctors would attribute a larger measure to reason, but a few of our respondents claimed to employ psychic powers in the examining room. An obstetrician told us, "I'm a born psychic. I realized it in the eighth grade, and I just forgot it, but it became obvious when I started visualizing future happenings. I can often predict what will happen with patients. I can't talk to anyone about this because it can get spooky, so I keep it to myself. I am able to see your body from your head to your toes and tell you what's medically wrong. A patient recently came in with a leg lesion, and I knew he also had liver problems as soon as he walked in. I told him he didn't eat properly because he was an alcoholic, and if he corrected that, his troubles would disappear. He was really impressed. His wife tells me that he stopped drinking and the problem with his leg went away."

This family doctor goes even further with esoteric diagnoses: "I talk to people's bodies, kinesthetically and telepathically. I might ask the liver how it's doing, and I get an answer, either a feeling or a vision. I work a lot with women who can't get pregnant. One woman in her late thirties hadn't been able to become pregnant for three or four years and was traumatized by all the drugs she had to take. I asked the spirit of the child who wanted to enter her body why it couldn't. The spirit replied, 'Because her pituitary isn't strong enough.'

"I told the patient, 'Here's what I believe, and you can accept it or not.' She appeared healthy, but I gave her pituitary supplements and herbs. Eventually I felt that her pituitary problem was corrected and the spirit was ready to enter. The patient got pregnant and is convinced that her child is a miracle."

Reflecting on such experiences, the doctor said: "You know, there's a part of me that is astounded by all of this. Yet, I can also feel very matter-of-fact about it and say, 'I don't think this is crazy at all.' I'm known to be intuitive, but my desire is to train my patients to trust their own body language."

DISEASE AS A SPIRITUAL LESSON

Finally, we hear from a general practitioner in Santa Monica who believes that disease should be viewed as a spiritual teacher: "I want the patient to learn from his illness. I have a saying, 'If you are unfortunate enough to have a disease, don't waste it. It can teach you a lot. And the worse a disease is, the more potential learning there is. I've had patients tell me their cancer had its positive aspects. Why? Because they came back to themselves. They had lost their way, and the cancer brought them back to what's important in life.

"Some modern-day diseases like Epstein-Barr virus and chronic fatigue syndrome may illustrate this. The way I see it, those illnesses derail people who have depleted themselves or gotten out of synch. Still they're working to keep up with their daily lives despite their body's warning them, 'Stop this!' So the Epstein-Barr virus becomes their rescuer. I tell them, 'Your symptoms are really horrible, but my spiritual view is that this is the best thing that ever happened to you and you'll be grateful because it's a messenger of change.' Of course, if they don't understand me, they may think, 'What a jerk! I'm suffering, my life's falling apart, and he's telling me it's the best thing that ever happened to me.'

"One patient did say something like that to me, so I asked her, 'What can't you do now that you have this virus?' She replied, 'I can't do anything. I have to eat only simple foods and can't overexert myself. I have to get to bed early and rest during the day.' I said, 'Is that bad? That's exactly what you've needed, but you haven't had the strength to ask for it. This virus is telling you to reorient your life.' "

CONCLUSIONS REGARDING THE SPIRITUAL DIMENSION

Beliefs must be tempered with hard facts and common sense. Ascribing a moral or spiritual subtext to an illness can be dangerous. If taken to an extreme, patients might forgo effective treatment because they believe it is God's will that they suffer, or because they feel they *must* go through the pain in order to ascertain the higher meaning of their illnesses. They might also succumb to feelings of inadequacy or shame, believing that their affliction is a payback for previous misdeeds or improper thoughts. History, unfortunately, has witnessed the disastrous effect of ascribing spiritual values to disease, such as when leprosy was regarded as proof of sin and justification for exile. Hearing certain demagogues rant about AIDS victims today makes leper colonies seem not so distant in time.

That having been said, it is also true that medical science cannot afford to ignore the evidence that spiritual factors play an important role in the onset and cure of disease. Almost anyone who is involved in medicine for any length of time can attest to the power of strongly held belief systems. Prayer and faith have long been known to relieve pain and suffering, and even, in certain remarkable instances, to bring about full recovery. Rational medicine has its own explanations of such phenomena—chance, suggestion, remission, etc.—but these might not be adequate. It could be argued that the fundamental premises of our rational-empirical tradition preclude a role for spirit and religion, that the two historical streams are destined never to cross paths. Nevertheless, the attempt must be made; phenomena such as those discussed in this chapter deserve further, serious examination. As Henry Sigerist's history of religious medicine concludes, "It is always present because it satisfies an ever-existing need."

CHAPTER 9

THE PUSH AND PULL OF CHANGE

Like all dynamic institutions, modern medicine is pushed and pulled by forces that both compel and resist change. The doctors we interviewed addressed many current problems that are in need of solutions. These include the spiraling cost of medical care, the administrative nightmare of third-party payment, the tragedy of uninsured patients, overspecialization and overreliance on technology, and the legal atmosphere that has doctors running scared and has sent malpractice insurance premiums soaring into the six-figure range. Our respondents added little that was fresh to the debate on these issues. Of considerable interest, however, was what they chose to say on the subject of innovation in medical practice. Many were outspoken about the forces that constrain creativity and inhibit the introduction of new ideas.

It should be noted that we included here only those accounts that were critical of the status quo. Naturally, these tended to come from doctors who are receptive to unconventional practices, a distinct but vocal minority. For the most part, our doctors believed that the institutional processes restraining inventive practices serve as important safeguards against charlatanry. However, the physicians you are about to hear from contend that the system is excessively inhibiting. "Sure, restraining mechanisms are necessary," said one. "But, we have to ask, to what extent are they repressive, inhibiting, and prohibitive? How can we strike a middle ground? Provisions should be made for innovative ideas to be tried, investigated, and readily shared, without penalizing doctors or jeopardizing patients."

HARDENING OF THE CATEGORIES

The most commonly mentioned inhibition to change was also the most obvious: what one New York physician characterized as "the normal inertia of human beings." He was referring to the tendency of his fellow physicians to protect the status quo and to do things strictly in accord with established customs: "We tend to move in a prescribed orbit. We don't easily break out of patterns of thought and behavior. Medicine *appears* to be progressive because we're always introducing new drugs and technologies. But that doesn't necessarily break down any boundaries.

"The innovations in medicine come from professional researchers, not so much the practicing physicians. Doctors are craftsmen who practice what others invent. The research people are the ones who push the frontiers, but most of them are Ph.D.s or doctors who left practice for the lab. Often they lack the practitioners' wisdom, which is gleaned from their clinical experience."

A Los Angeles pediatrician expressed the problem this way: "Training is by the book. We're not taught to be innovative, we're taught to go by the operating manual, like a pilot who has to go through a prescribed series of steps before flying a plane. You try to eliminate all guessing and not stray from the customary."

The same doctor was also eager to point out that many physicians who think of themselves as the vanguard can be just as hidebound as the conservatives they decry: "You look at the so-called holistic crowd. They pay lip service to treating the 'whole person,' but then a patient comes in and they give him an herb instead of a drug, or acupuncture instead of physical therapy, or whatever. Are they really treating the whole person? They're just following someone else's precept, albeit an unorthodox one.

"The point is, there are conservatives and progressives in every camp. Some of the holistic practices are as old as Hippocrates. So, is it progressive or reactionary? Is a mainstream doctor who tries the latest drug progressive or reactionary? A lot of the holistic group imitate each other. They're faddish. I'm not saying what they're doing isn't effective. I'm saying they can be just as rigid, just as ideological, just as stuck as the mainstream crowd. And in some cases they're just as elitist and just as exclusionary. It's the same tunnel vision, only looking down a different tunnel."

Treatments rooted in theories that run counter to mainstream thought meet the greatest resistance. Even when, in practice, a treatment proves to be efficacious, it might be discounted simply because no one can explain *why* it works. History records many such instances: the use of colchicum to treat gout, for example. Here a San Diego doctor explains why some of the methods he favors have not caught on despite achieving good results:

"It's a question of familiarity. If you tell a doctor that a patient with chronic colitis or an ulcer can be treated by working on acupuncture meridians, he's going to look at you as if you're a quack. When I tell physicians about my success rate, they look at me as if I'm bragging or lying. Our doctors are trained to see the body as comprised of various systems, not like the Eastern approach where the body is viewed as an entity in and of itself. Disease develops because of a blockage in the flow of energy, and when you remove the block, the body will heal itself.

"I attended a conference last summer, and the lecturer on back pain was an eminent orthopedic surgeon. He said basically the same thing I heard when I was an orthopedic resident ten years ago. So I asked him, 'What about chiropractic manipulation? What about alternative forms of treatment?' His response was, 'None of them have been shown to produce long-term benefits.' I laughed, because I'm convinced that millions of patients have gotten sustained relief from acupuncture, chiropractic, and osteopathy.

"After I've treated a patient a few times for back pain and he has no pain a year later, no one can tell me that that patient was not helped by the treatment. Yet, a doctor will say that the patient would have gotten better anyway, or he really didn't have a problem, or it was the suggestion of telling him he was going to get better. That burns me up."

Some doctors believed that the aversion to change can be so strong that unorthodox practitioners run a serious risk of being ostracized by their peers. One said she was censured when she began advocating a controversial method of diagnosis and treatment: "There were times at meetings when there was a vacuum around me. Everybody would have somebody sitting on both sides of them except me. When I went to the hospital, my few friends would signal for me to come into their office and would then quickly shut the door so no one could see that they were talking to me."

She attempted to vindicate herself with careful research: "I did double-blind studies showing that the treatment worked. But when I went to publish the articles, I couldn't get them into the journals. The journals, of course, are edited by doctors who are specialists in drugs, and their research is subsidized by the drug industry. Why would they publish something about a method that has nothing to do with drugs? They always find something wrong. I even took movies of patients, and the editors said they were acting. I did blood studies. They were unacceptable. I showed brain wave changes. They said I didn't have enough controls. I finally said, 'Forget it. They're never going to believe me.' "

While she retained her faculty position, she says her status was diminished: "I was no longer allowed to teach the medical students or asked to give the board examinations. I once had a lot of credibility. But all of a sudden, when I said, 'I believe these methods work,' I was no longer credible."

IMPATIENT PATIENTS

According to several doctors, patients can be just as conservative as physicians, sometimes even more so. Because a person in distress takes comfort in the familiar, doctors say they have to use discretion when recommending an unconventional treatment. "Some patients freak out if you do something beyond the pale," said an internist whose repertoire ranges far afield. "You go too far and you lose patients. Then they go to the next doctor and make you sound weirder than you really are. Most people want the reassurance of a prescription or a shot—the things their family doctor did when they were kids and got sick."

One unconventional doctor said that many patients resist her suggestions because they require an investment of time or energy: "It's a shame, but modern medicine has promulgated this notion that the patient's participation ends when he shows up at the hospital or takes his medicine on time. A lot of the methods that I consider new and exciting put greater responsibility into the patient's hands. If you believe that healing works best when patients are involved, if you believe they will be healthier longer if they take more responsibility for themselves, if you want them to sit and meditate instead of taking a tranquilizer, or you give them some herbs that might take a few extra days to work but without any side effects, you're asking the patient to actively cooperate. Many of them prefer to be passive. If they could drop off their bodies at your office like they drop off their car at their mechanic's, they'd be happier."

Two doctors who use unorthodox methods reported that some of their colleagues, who are also their patients, are reluctant to refer their own patients because of their concern for their reputations. Said a Philadelphia-based pain specialist: "I can't tell you how many colleagues of mine have come to me for acupuncture and biofeedback. They know what I do works. But do they send me patients? Only after everything else fails. Why? They don't want to lose their respectability. They're covering their ass, so they can say they sent the patient to an orthopedist or whatever, and they tried the latest FDA-approved pain medication. But, when *they're* in pain, they come right to me. They don't waste any time."

A Los Angeles doctor who is outspoken in his preference for alternative medicine concurs: "A lot of doctors come to me as patients and specifically ask for acupuncture. Now, they never refer *their* patients to me for acupuncture. They send them to a neurosurgeon, neurologist, or an orthopedist. If those doctors are unsuccessful, *then* they send the patients to me. But the *doctor* comes straight to me. They're afraid that if they refer someone to me right off the bat, then it looks like they approve of what I do."

THE BOTTOM LINE OF MEDICINE

Over and above the human tendency to resist new ideas or methods are a number of economic and legal restraints. Their impact has reached all facets of medicine. One aspect that was mentioned frequently is the trend toward "cost-effective practice."

"If you're trying to maximize the number of patients you see," contends a general practitioner in Santa Barbara, "it encourages conservative practice. Reaching out of bounds takes time. You have to find sources that don't come to you in the mail. You have to read, to speak to other docs, to think. Also, alternative procedures usually entail giving more time to the patient. There is more to explain, more questions to ask, more hands-on things to do, all of which take time. That means you can squeeze in fewer paid office visits in the day."

A cardiologist who uses psychotherapy as an adjunct to traditional practices agrees: "I see a patient for an hour. The initial screening is an hour and a half to two. That's very different from other cardiologists, who spend maybe fifteen minutes with a patient. If you're paid per visit and you spend twice as much time with a patient, you make half as much money. Plus, many things I can do to help a patient won't be reimbursed by the insurance companies. Personally, I can't practice any other way, but I can understand why someone with a family to support can't do what I do."

Third-party medicine—wherein an outside agency, not the patient, is responsible for reimbursement—has transformed not only the economics of medicine but the way it is practiced. A Boston pain specialist addressed this issue: "Society actually discourages preventive medicine because the insurance companies don't pay for it. They encourage treatment and testing once the disease process occurs, and doctors and patients tend to compound the problem. It's very easy to give codeine to patients with back pain, and they *want* codeine. The alternative—starting a patient on a series of treatments—requires much more of your and the patient's time."

Complained a Denver general practitioner: "We not only have to spend an incredible amount of time filling out forms, and a lot of money paying for clerical help, but we are now told exactly what treatments are acceptable for which diagnoses. The insurers identify the diagnosis by code and tell you exactly how much they will pay. It doesn't foster creativity. It virtually takes the art out of doctoring. You're locked into a pretty limited selection."

A family doctor in the San Francisco area spoke to the same issue: "I think there is an increasing demand for accredited training and responsible practice of complementary techniques. But private insurance policies are incredibly expensive, and most HMOs refuse to cover those procedures. So there are fewer insurance-backed patients to receive these services and very few physicians who can afford to use labor-intensive procedures. So, there are obstacles to satisfy what seems to be a growing demand."

WHO WILL PAY FOR RESEARCH?

Several physicians described a Catch-22 situation: only procedures whose effectiveness is backed by rigorous testing can hope to gain acceptance (even though there is not enough "outcome research" to prove what works over time), but unorthodox treatments are not as likely to be studied in the first place. "In order to do a really good study, you need money and resources," said a Los Angeles physician who has several small research projects he'd like to pursue. "I see treatments that work in my practice, and I'm told, 'Go ahead and investigate them.' How? Where? You can't just do some informal study. You have to do a full-blown research protocol or no one will pay attention. I'd have to give up my practice and apply for a grant. Writing grant proposals and locating agencies that might consider them can be a full-time job.

"The other way ideas get studied is if they promise to produce a profit. Major companies that manufacture drugs or high-tech equipment are not going to fund research for some alternative concepts that may compete with their products. That's why you don't see any experiments on vitamins and minerals or nutritional remedies and herbs—you can't patent those things, so there's no incentive for a private company to study them. However, pharmaceutical companies have successfully lobbied the FDA to issue restrictions on the labeling of those items. In a few years, they will be unable to state that they aid in any form of healing."

A few doctors also claimed that pharmaceutical companies work to prevent others from doing research on alternative treatments. Says an internist whose practice draws on Chinese and Indian traditions: "I don't think the drug industry has been entirely forthright in all its promotions and statements. They have tremendous wealth behind them and they perceive as a threat anything beyond their purview. I don't know if they directly lobby against alternatives, but certainly the way they promote their own products works against their acceptance. Take stress reduction. Pills are no answer to reducing stress, but you see promotions for pills that reduce stress. Also, there is the matter of research funding. You won't see Hoffman-LaRoche, which makes Valium, do research on meditation."

A family physician in Chicago believes that the pharmaceutical

industry conspires to suppress information about nutritional therapies: "It costs a minimum of fifteen million dollars to test a drug,
sometimes up to a hundred million for the animal experimentation
and double-blind studies required by the FDA. This means that only
patentable substances will have a sponsor. The drug companies that
spend money to develop patentable drugs subsidize the medical journals. If an editor of a medical journal is inclined to publish articles
about nutrition, the drug companies are not likely to buy ad space in
that journal."

It should be noted that in July 1992, the National Institutes of
Health established an Office for the Study of Unconventional Medical
Practices. It was the first time government funds had been allocated
for scientific research on alternative treatments. At the time this book
was completed, no results had yet been obtained.

STAYING OUT OF TROUBLE

Physicians are also restrained from prescribing unorthodox treatments
by the threats of lawsuits, censure by medical authorities, or even
criminal action. Says a G.P. in Orange County, California: "The
atmosphere is so litigious, you have to think about malpractice suits
all the time. If you want to try something you think might work and
that you know is harmless, you have to think twice. What if something
does happen and the patient blames it on the treatment. What if
nothing happens and they sue you because you didn't prescribe the
standard procedure? That's why you see doctors sending patients for
every test imaginable and to every specialist imaginable, regardless of
the cost. If you don't check out one possible diagnosis because you
think it's unlikely, you open yourself up to a lawsuit."

In addition to potential lawsuits from disgruntled patients, doctors
who extend the boundaries of their practice run the risk of censure
from the authorities that police the profession. Anyone who deviates
from community standards of practice and behavior can become a

pariah or even lose his license. From our respondents we heard no fewer than four such tales. We relate them here from the doctors' points of view. First, an Oregon physician with a long history on the frontier:

"I was told that anybody who wasn't an M.D. was a quack. But I found that chiropractors and naturopaths often had good results, sometimes even better than what medical doctors were getting, and cheaper and safer. But I made a mistake by working with them. I'd oversee their work and sign the insurance papers under my name. I didn't keep any of the money because I hadn't performed the services directly. But the insurance companies called the Board of Medical Examiners, and the board said that was malfeasance. They told me to surrender my license. They said if I refused they'd drag me through the mud and put my name in the paper and embarrass me. So my wife said, 'Just dump it. You're about ready to retire anyway.' So I did. I don't practice anymore."

The doctor believes that the action against him was a vendetta for a career of outspoken opinions: "If I were an ordinary, regular doctor, they would have simply said, 'Don't do this.' But they thought I was still a loose cannon, and in a way they were right. The board needs to be sure that medical doctors practice the way they're supposed to: make a diagnosis, treat it with a drug. So, I have no ill feeling toward them, except I think they overdid it with me. I wasn't a drunk. I didn't take drugs. I had a good reputation. But they felt I was not the kind of doctor they wanted to encourage."

Another unconventional physician has been jousting with the authorities since 1974: "It started with laetrile. Laetrile is a nutritional product containing benzaldehyde and other ingredients—apricot seeds, apple seeds, lentils, lima beans. It was commercially produced in Germany. It seemed to help cancer patients by increasing their appetite and decreasing pain. It also improved their mood and helped them gain weight. So I started using it with a cancer patient, to help reduce her pain. There were only a few of us using it then, and we got into trouble because the Board of Medical Examiners said it couldn't be used as a cancer treatment. Only chemotherapy, radiation, and surgery are legal treatments. We said we *weren't* using it as a cancer treatment. We were using it as a nutritional supplement for pain, appetite, and mood. I believe the drug companies just don't want nutritional remedies, unless they have to be prescribed."

While he was ultimately pardoned for the laetrile charge, the doctor's problems persisted. An investigator posing as a patient filed charges against him for using what were termed improper diagnostic procedures. He was put on probation, but later cleared when a judge ruled that he had been a victim of discriminatory prosecution.

A Northern California veteran of alternative medicine said: "I was censored by the medical staff at the hospital. I had been using Vitamin C and Vitamin E postoperatively, and the patients did extremely well. They healed promptly, and their hospitalization was short. Well, I got flak from the hospital. They said that it wasn't approved, it was dangerous, it might cause kidney stones, and we might get sued. Now, I've given massive doses of Vitamin C to over seventeen thousand people without a single case of kidney stones.

"Those of us who would like to be more creative in our practices live with a certain degree of anxiety that the board is going to come down on us. I think the majority of charges brought against physicians are for drug addiction, insurance fraud, sexual abuse of patients, and matters like that, which the board is supposed to protect against. But some of the most severe penalties have been dealt out for transgressions such as aiding and abetting a chiropractor or using Vitamin A in infected children.

"Sure, you're going to have some quackery, and there are bound to be some difficulties, but I think that in the long run we'd all be much better off if doctors had more leeway. I think that the risk posed by those few doctors who might take advantage of that freedom would be insignificant compared to the damage done by conservatism."

At the time of our interview, the next physician was in the midst of a battle to keep his license: "The state has seen fit to charge me with incompetence because I include nutritional medicine in my practice. The charges against me are rather broad. They have listed all the things I do, things I'm proud of, and have called them medically unnecessary or medically unindicated. I've been charged with fraud, incompetence, and negligence. Now, to me, fraud means you're doing something strictly for the money and that you know in your heart is worthless. I'm clearly not doing that.

"I've been under scrutiny for nine years, and in all that time, the only patient complaint they could dig up was a woman who requested her records and the records had been lost. I think I'm being used as a political football. It's a thinly veiled attempt to prevent freedom of choice by patients who prefer alternative practices. I think I'm going to prevail after a long, arduous, expensive process."

While they have not been brought up on charges, several doctors we interviewed said they felt intimidated by actions taken against their colleagues. Indeed, some feel that such intimidation is precisely the result authorities have in mind. One Santa Monica G.P. explained his view: "I gave up a lot of alternative methods when my friend got burned by the board. I wanted to keep myself as straight as I could because I didn't want to go through the same thing. I didn't want to fight, because everyone I know who fights organized medicine ends up with their license taken away, or in jail."

A Massachusetts physician concurs: "There is tremendous emphasis placed on standard of care. There are a lot of things that I might be tempted to try, but I would never do them because they don't fall within those standards. You can get into trouble. The worst would be a malpractice suit against you, and the least would be that the quality assurance board would slap you on the hands and say, 'What the hell are you doing?' The other day, a lady came in with an acutely swollen tongue. It looked like an allergic reaction, and my colleague told her to swish some epinephrine around in her mouth. Now, epinephrine is good for acute allergic reactions, but it's usually given subcutaneously; however, he decided to give it to her as a mouth wash. I'm sure it worked, but I wouldn't do that because it's not the standard of care."

THE INEVITABILITY OF CHANGE

Despite the many psychological and institutional restraints on innovation, medicine has always been a dynamic system. It has always been characterized by change, and it always will change, as long as there are individuals who question assumptions and challenge orthodoxy—and as long as the advocates of change are prepared to submit their ideas to the test of scientific experimentation.

In the long run, the wheat will be separated from the chaff and the boundaries of medicine will be expanded. More than likely, however, the principal force to compel the evolution of medicine will be the marketplace. A Los Angeles cardiologist expressed this view compellingly: "If patients approach health care the way they approach buying a car or a VCR, by becoming well-informed consumers, making their complaints heard, demanding variety and quality, then change will happen. Without that, you'll have to wait for governments and the medical establishment to do this, and that could be a long wait."

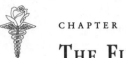

CHAPTER 10

THE FUTURE OF MEDICINE

Like many Americans, the doctors in our sample expressed concern about the present state of medicine. Faced with heightened expectations and demands for answers to vexing health-oriented social and ethical problems, they spoke of the urgent need to define their role and create workable guidelines for the problems they face daily, such as the system of third-party payments, with its burden of paperwork and red tape; the more than thirty-seven million Americans who do not have health insurance; the extraordinary cost of ordinary health care and catastrophic illness; the need for a more equitable way to adjudicate malpractice suits, to raise the quality of hospital and nursing-home care, develop appropriate facilities for the terminally ill, and improve public health education.

Perhaps because our interviews centered on the treatment room, our respondents, while expressing an awareness of the problems at hand, offered few novel solutions to matters of public policy that have been closely examined in a number of recent books and articles. However, one subject that seemed close to their hearts was the training of physicians. Virtually every doctor we interviewed had something to say about this, and their opinions seemed to cut across ideological lines. Most of their remarks centered on the need to cultivate those human qualities we would like our doctors to have.

One general practitioner provided a quite jaundiced characterization of an office visit: "I'm concerned about the loss of human dignity in medical practice. Medicine requires a certain gentility and respect for people. A doctor's office should be a place of refuge from pain and trouble, but it's becoming a mockery. The waiting room is usually uninviting in its impersonal design, and is typically filled with people, like an overbooked hotel. The average doctor often sees many more patients than he should, but not as many as need his care. If it's a first visit, you are given a long, tedious form to fill out by a diffident office worker, and the emphasis generally is, 'How are you going to pay for your treatment?' Finally, you're ushered into another room, where you get the false notion that you're being taken care of, but it's really another depot where you sit on a cold stool in a slit-back gown and contemplate your fate. Periodically, the nurse peeks in and tells you the doctor will be with you momentarily.

"Finally, he comes in, and he's harassed and busy. He sits down, opens your file, and scans it to remind himself who you are. You get a once-over, after which he might prescribe some pills or send you to someone else for additional tests. If you're lucky, you may get a chance to see him in his inner sanctum for a brief period. Nowadays, you can even answer a huge questionnaire and get a computer printout with a diagnosis. What's next? Maybe people should have those product bars on them so we can run the wand over them like in a supermarket. Then we'd have everything we need to know about them. It's certainly not a caring environment, even for a well patient being seen for a routine exam.

"If that type of atmosphere is going to change, it has to start with medical school, maybe even pre-med. We have to get properly motivated, well-rounded people into the field and train them to be humane as well as technically competent."

In a similar vein, a young family doctor expressed a certain disillusionment: "I'm frustrated by the absence of humanity in medical practice. I went to medical school because I was idealistic. I wanted to be part of this great institution where everyone worked together to make people's lives easier. I figured there would be teachers to admire and emulate, but something dies inside many students while in training. They get all caught up in the competition, and the competition obscures their idealism.

"I see too many doctors coming out of training who are preoccupied with making money and enhancing their egos, not the joy of healing people. I realize that most of them enter practice with tens of thousands of dollars of debt due to the cost of their training, but that should not negate their passion for helping people. Most of them start out as caring individuals, but the process can beat it out of them. It's not as sustaining, in the short run, to be compassionate as it is to be acquisitive. When you get tired and worn out, being a humanitarian is not immediately fulfilling.

"Medical education has to work more from a human standpoint than a technological standpoint. It's getting so mechanized, so impersonal. If the doctor comes into the room with empathy and understanding, the patient is going to get well faster than if the doctor is aloof. This ability to identify with what the patient is feeling, to really listen, is crucial. By providing the patient with an empathetic doctor as his ally, you have begun the healing process."

ON WHO GOES TO MEDICAL SCHOOL

Because we selected the most expressive and provocative doctors' statements, their overall tone is perhaps more emotionally charged than the majority. However, their comments are, in spirit, consistent with the views of most respondents who answered the question, "What would you do if you were put in charge of medical training?"

Several would-be reformers said they would begin the process with the pre-med curriculum and medical school admissions policies. One doctor said, "I would argue for a broader exposure to the humanities in pre-med. I would want students who had literature and history courses as opposed to all science. Today, the entering medical student most commonly has a degree in chemistry or biology, but traditionally, most of the leading family physicians, internists, and surgeons were well educated beyond their medical studies.

"What I see too often are pre-med students who try to get the best grades in science courses while ignoring the fields of fine arts, humanities, social sciences, and history. You learn what makes people tick through a variety of down-to-earth life experiences—even being a patient yourself. I think you have to be well rounded and well read, so you can talk to all kinds of people. I suppose it's just easier for admissions committees to emphasize science and grade-point averages. It's a lot harder for them to sit down with someone and decide after an interview whether the applicant is going to make a good physician. I would pick students who have an interest in people, mastered an art, traveled, and, in general, had experiences that would help them become well integrated people, rather than eggheads who made straight A's in biochemistry."

Several physicians said they would pay closer attention to the psychological traits of potential doctors: "I think personality factors should be evaluated as part of entry to med school. I once served on the admissions committee of a prominent medical school. When I interviewed candidates, I wanted to learn something about their general character. I'd try to ask fairly pointed questions about their attitudes and beliefs, but I was warned by the administrators, who thought it was an unwarranted intrusion. So, I couldn't get a good appraisal of their personalities. In addition to determining their motivation, intelligence, and maturity, it would be desirable to know how close the applicant fits the profile of what we assume the 'ideal doctor' to be. This would certainly include a consideration of their ethical and moral values, as might well be required for applicants to the ministry, and perhaps for politicians as well."

ON THE NEED TO CHANGE THE CURRICULUM

Almost all our doctors called for changes in the medical school curriculum. Those changes mentioned most often entailed less classroom work and basic science, with more emphasis on hands-on experience:

"I would like to see an expansion of the educational base that the doctor stands on. An educated person in the broad sense is better equipped to enter the profession of healing than the narrow technological wizard. Unfortunately, the highest priority is given to proficiency in scientific and technical skills, and the lowest priority is the humanities. Nowadays, many doctors are so enamored of technology that they neglect all the other factors that go into healing.

"There's too much emphasis on mathematics. The only time I've ever used it is to figure out my income taxes. The little bit we use in everyday practice you can get in the ninth grade. Sure, those doctors who go into research need it, but only a certain type of person is good at it, and they don't necessarily make the best doctors.

"I'm concerned that with all the emphasis on technology and computer-based diagnosis we might fool ourselves into thinking we can eliminate the human touch. Of course we should safeguard against fallibility, but there are things our minds bring to medicine that no machine can hope to duplicate. A big part of medical diagnosis is intuition. You get hunches, you sense things. We should look for ways to enhance our intuitive abilities."

In that regard several doctors believed the curriculum should do more to develop creative thinking: "Medical training would benefit enormously by including courses designed to improve creative thinking and problem solving rather than the current emphasis on rote memory and the regurgitation of facts.

"Students should be taught how to trust their own powers of observation and to have the confidence that their perceptions are valid and important—not only because they can offer more to the evaluation of a particular patient but because their insights might lead to a beneficial discovery."

In regard to training, other doctors would choose to broaden the perspectives of future doctors to embrace the social context of medicine. One physician articulated his personal thesis regarding physician education:

"There should be more emphasis on ways of understanding the relationship between people and communities. What effects do a city's pollution and homeless population have on the health of its citizens? What impact will be made by the growing number of geriatric patients? Medical students should study the socio-cultural implications of health care, which may include patients' attitudes about nutrition, birth control, and sex practices. Doctors need to be aware that patients from various cultures often express their symptoms and responses to illnesses in different terms and mannerisms than were described in medical texts. They must learn how to interpret these descriptions in order to make proper diagnoses.

"Physicians should also be knowledgeable of the vast scope and interrelationships of the economics of medicine. How do community health clinics, substance-abuse centers, and AIDS hospices, or their absence, impact a community's taxes and overall services? Certainly medical prevention is more cost-effective than medical treatment and results in more revenue for other community services, such as parks and schools. Physicians need to know how and where to refer patients who require special medical services and those patients who are victims of rape or physical abuse and may be suffering with Post Traumatic Syndrome. Every major medical question is a political question: who gets it, who pays for it, who has the power to determine the shape of the delivery system, who has access to it? These are political questions, and physicians should be prepared to think about them.

"In addition to their medical studies, they should be taught business management skills and how to deal with those outside forces that impact the daily operation of their practices: the legal system, bureau-

crats, governmental agencies, insurance companies and all the regula-
tions, and how to police their own quality assurance. All these are
basic issues, and they weren't part of my medical training.

"I would also have them study community medicine—how to be
involved in the community they practice in and to work with the
people with respect to social services and public-health issues. On the
individual level, doctors should be trained to involve the patient more
in the decision making. I think we spend too much time focusing on
diagnosis and technology and not enough time on patient involvement
and participation in the community."

An industrial psychiatrist pointed out that medical training ignores
a vital aspect of patients' lives: their occupations. "So many people
have work-related problems, whether it's stress or anxiety from working in a boring, repetitive job, or from the pressures of a competitive,
unappreciated career. The nature of people's work has a tremendous
impact on their health. Doctors should understand these things. We
should at least be knowledgeable of the hazards of various occupations. I had a patient with hypertension and ulcers. It turned out that
he was unhappy and depressed; he hated his job, but he couldn't quit
because he's got three kids, a mortgage, the whole enchilada. What am
I supposed to do? I can make him feel better, but how long will it last
when he's got to go back to the same job that's making him ill?
Sometimes I feel like the trainer in a boxer's corner. I get one minute
between rounds to fix him up, and then the bell sounds and he has to
go back into the ring and get beaten up again. Plato believed that the
highest goal a person could attain was to do the work he was happiest
in. We need a more comprehensive way to psychologically match
people to jobs."

Perhaps the one idea that was mentioned more than any other was
to involve students with patients much earlier in their training:

"When I went to medical school, the first two years were filled with
textbooks and classroom lectures presented in the most boring teaching format imaginable. Only in our third and fourth years did we begin

to do clinical work. I think that you have to start with native curiosity, with wanting to know the answers to questions. A lot of that inquisitiveness is integrated through clinical experiences. After you've seen someone with hepatitis, then the classroom distinctions between different kinds of hepatitis, and the different viruses that cause them, become much more meaningful. The way medical students have traditionally been taught, I feel, has been with too much rote memorization in the first two years, with little or no exposure to patients."

That opinion was mirrored by many, such as this New England internist: "They take students, some with a pretty decent liberal arts education, and turn them into quasi-scientists. Everybody has to prepare for the boards, and the last time I looked they didn't have any social questions on them. They were strictly classroom and laboratory issues. It really wasn't that applicable to daily clinical practice.

"They teach as if medicine is a scientific study exclusively, when it should also be a study of the biosocial relationships of human beings in health and disease. You're taught a lot that has very little relevance for treating patients. You're taught about obscure pathological tests and treatments, which are always left to specialists anyway. Why not trade that time in for something more real, like helping a patient deal with being depressed over his illness or being away from his job or kids?

"We spend weeks and weeks on laboratory work—microbiology, and embryology, and tissue cultures and all that. It's dead weight. I never spent a minute on it after I left school. A passing familiarity would be sufficient for most doctors. The sad thing is, a lot of students with the soul of a doctor are weeded out because they're not superior in subjects like chemistry or physics. Have you ever seen that British TV show, 'All Creatures Great and Small,' about veterinarians? Those animals got the kind of treatment that humans ought to be getting."

Another respondent had this practical suggestion: "I would start everybody out as an emergency medical technician. They would get some background, some place to categorize the information that they're going to be getting. My biggest frustration was that they threw all these diseases at us and we didn't have any way to really organize it. It didn't fit anywhere. I wanted to know how to take care of people. There wasn't anything to hang a hat on. I think you should put students out in the field and teach them CPR and rescue techniques, and have them go with the ambulances to where the ground zero of medicine lies.

"Do that for six months. Then, when they come back, they'll know why they have to learn about basic science and anatomy. They've seen pathology in action that is relevant to what they're learning and that gives them a frame of reference. It will all come naturally, and they'll learn how to cope with acute stress and injury. Plus, it would help staff emergency rooms.

"I think the medical schools want to be purists—you know, start with the basic building blocks and work your way up. You just can't take in all that information without some reference point. Usually, you get some clinical exposure in your second year—how to do a physical examination. You start seeing patients in your third year. Much of the time is spent in basically boring, repetitious book learning. Personally, I was tired of book learning when I got out of college."

This Los Angeles family practitioner had a similar view: "I would have medical students spend less time in the hospital, where there's all that technology and an extraordinarily sick population, and I'd put them in community clinics. That way they'd be exposed early on to the kind of patients they will be seeing in their careers. I would put them where they're likely to see a wide variety of everyday illnesses. Right now, the only time doctors get to see those things is if they do a family practice residency. Otherwise, they are not exposed to them until the day they open their practices.

"I would also make sure that residents got more experience in out-patient settings. As interns, we had half a day a week in an out-patient clinic, and even in the third year I believe it was only one and a half days. I remember being frustrated—not enough patients, not enough hands-on experience, and teachers who were hard to find when you wanted to ask a question. By giving them more exposure to out-patient care, they would be equipped to deal with situations they will actually face in their day-to-day activities."

Some physicians were critical of the medical school faculty, emphasizing their role as examples to the next generation of doctors: "It's important for students to have role models who deeply care about patients and are competent and intelligent. We really didn't see that enough. I remember the clinician who didn't give a damn about how people felt and the brilliant diagnostician who talked mostly to himself. But students should know that competence and compassion are not mutually exclusive. I look at the doctors that come out today as excellent technicians, but who don't know enough about people.

"I would want the professors to speak to the students' hearts, not just their heads. That is generally deficient in all medical schools. You're dealing with the brightest kids in the world. They're devoting twelve or more of the best years of their lives. When they come out, their enthusiasm and idealism has suffered. It's a grueling sort of ritual.

"I think the student-teacher relationship acts as a role model and reflects the way a student will be with his or her patients. Maybe it's a question of choosing the right faculty. I mean, doctors train doctors, so you're cloning yourselves generation after generation. Frankly, a lot of doctors shouldn't be on the faculty. A lot of them are focused on research and not well suited for teaching."

The subject of medical ethics came up in several contexts. This cardiologist would have future doctors think about philosophical issues as students: "I would get them to consider difficult questions about patient care. How do you make the tough decisions about who lives and who dies? How long someone should be on a respirator? What is brain-dead? You have to start thinking about those realities. And things like organ transplants, abortion, human experimentation, and genetic engineering—all these hot issues that they're going to have to deal with should be discussed in depth while they're learning to care for people. Doctors should be ethically trained. Whatever their judgments finally are, they should know why they got to those positions and how."

Apropros the main thrust of this book, a large number of doctors called for expanding the medical curriculum to cover methods now on the fringe.

"I would open the curriculum to other modalities. An elective here or there is not nearly enough. We just scratch the surface. We should be teaching treatment methods with no side effects as a first resort, not as a last resort. And I would give a whole course, maybe two courses, on the side effects of drugs, surgery and hospitalization, so doctors would be more self-critical.

"My medical school was a top school, but we did two years of pharmacology and only one optional hour of nutrition. I would make sure that everyone's trained in nutrition. And there should be a high priority on working with people about self-care and prevention. I'd give courses on Chinese medicine. I'd also provide instruction in caring for the dying, so that terminally ill patients would be treated better. I'd want to have a department of energy medicine, a department of psychoneuroimmunology, and a department of herbal medicine.

"Not that students have to become experts in all these modalities while they're in medical school, but they should be made aware that these things exist and that they are valid. The standard attitude is that if we haven't taught it to you, then it doesn't exist or it's quackery. We're making minuscule efforts to prepare our physicians for the twenty-first century. I think there will be many changes in health care, and physicians are going to have to integrate them into their practices somehow.

"I already see the consumer putting tremendous pressure on medical education to be sensitive to their needs. I would tell students that the patients they're going to see will want more natural forms of health care. There is a groundswell. You have no idea how many patients go to doctors and say, 'I found this in a health food store,' or 'I read about this in *Prevention* magazine,' or 'My masseur told me about this.' Patients should be encouraged to discuss those options with their doctors."

When asked what he would do if he were put in charge of a medical school, this Seattle physician said, "I'd be in seventh heaven! I felt my training was lacking. I think early on in med school there should be exposure to broad areas of healing, to give more attention to what else is out there. It's about time we incorporated a global view of healing, to make sure physicians are trained not only in allopathic medicine but in biofeedback, homeopathy, in acupuncture, and manipulation. The same treatments don't work for everyone. The fourth year of med school is all electives. I'd give them all these options so they can choose. I would emphasize the basics: nutrition, prevention, and general wellness, as opposed to disease processes."

ON THE NEED TO HUMANIZE TRAINING

In recent years, the question of whether aspects of medical training are excessively demanding has attracted considerable debate. On one side are critics who use terms such as harsh, brutal, and inhuman to describe the training process. They believe that too many potentially good doctors are lost to burnout and that many survivors emerge from their rigors exhausted and somewhat callous. On the other side are those who feel that the men and women responsible for our health, who are called upon to respond to emergencies under difficult conditions, should endure a trial by fire lest they be ill-prepared. It is difficult to say where our 250 doctors stood on the issue because it was not raised explicitly. However, so many chose to address it on their own that we can only surmise that the demands of medical training are a major concern. What follows are statements that represent the opinions of those critical of the process:

"In a profession where qualities like compassion and empathy and maturity should be the highest priorities, we hardly pay any attention to the students' psychological development. I don't know that we can train people to be compassionate, but I'm sure we can do a better job than we do, and we certainly shouldn't make things worse. But we lose a lot of the more sensitive students. I'm not sure you need to run around for twenty-four hours and even forty-eight hours at a time in order to learn medicine.

"I'd encourage students and residents to meet in informal groups and keep tabs on themselves, to support each other instead of competing with each other, because it can be so difficult going through it. We had a group that was so stressed out by the demands of the program and so angry at the indifference of our teachers that we used to meet at someone's apartment every week. We felt the need to bolster each other to help us get through it with our sanity. It didn't last very long, though, because the sense of competition won out."

A female family physician in Philadelphia called for more humane hours in residency: "The model that has existed for many decades in this country is that of a male physician who devotes most of his waking hours to the practice of medicine and is backed up by a wife who does all the parenting and keeps the household running. The ideal they strive for is to devote the maximum number of hours possible to medicine to the virtual exclusion of personal interests and family responsibilities. I think the training model is related to that. It makes you think that this is what you have to do for the rest of your life.

"I disagree with that. As a model, it's outdated. It makes physicians one-dimensional. The grind of residency puts you under a huge amount of pressure, physically and emotionally. It can be so grueling that we damage or lose a lot of the best, most humane, most brilliant physicians. The unimpaired are not necessarily gifted, but they have the wherewithal to get through the obstacle course of training."

This general practitioner concurred, calling for more support systems for doctors in training: "The first thing I would do is train physicians to take care of their own health, because that's the last thing they learn, if they ever learn it at all. When I came out of training, I was a physical and mental wreck. Maybe it's better now than when I was going through it, but I still read about residents who are doing endless hours on duty. By the time they're finished, some doctors are totally burned out and dehumanized. I would teach them how to survive, and I would teach them to practice in a way that they could get satisfaction out of it.

"I think nine out of ten people who are attracted to medicine are empathic, caring, feeling people, and it's a shame that some of these qualities get diminished by the ordeal of training. They lose some of the human qualities that attracted them to medicine in the first place.

"There also seems to be a taboo against being an individual in medicine, and it's reinforced in the medical school experience. It used to be that the practitioner's art was an important thing, but now it seems that to survive training you have to conform and give up some of the sensibility that makes for creative individuals. Schools seem to be trying to produce a formula model of a doctor."

Several doctors felt that medical training should focus more on psychological and emotional development. One veteran of private practice and medical school faculties put it this way: "We should screen future doctors more carefully in the course of their training. Are there ways to predict who will be ethical, responsible, and honest? Who will have good bedside manners? We can't do it with precision, the way you can teach someone to use a stethoscope. But there is much more we can do. We have to be more attuned to the student's psychological makeup.

"I would have every intern and resident interviewed by a person posing as a patient, as a kind of quality control, as a teaching device. I'd have a course on medical etiquette—all about how to be a caring human being. There should be a way for doctors to check themselves on those qualities, just as they check for whether they're diagnosing and prescribing correctly. Self-knowledge should be encouraged—social skills, human decency, and understanding. Patients are very sensitive to these things. Certain personality characteristics go against the grain of good doctoring, and we should watch out for them during training and do more to help those people.

"At one point in my career, I was in charge of residency training. There was a very strong sense that you should not meddle in the personal aspects of how doctors feel and what makes them tick. There's a lot of resistance to it. Unless the doctor elects to go into psychotherapy, that aspect of his life is totally ignored. Any kind of emotional training is not encouraged, even on an elective basis. I tried to get medical students together informally, in a kind of group interchange, but the dean made me stop. He was worried that a student might get upset during a session and get a bad grade or whatever and sue the school because it was the group sessions that screwed him up. So it is out of bounds. You can't get into their emotional lives unless they have a breakdown, and if they do, they may become pariahs."

Another perspective on this was provided by a San Francisco internist: "We should take a page out of the training for psychotherapists. They know that what's going on in their own hearts and minds can affect how they work with their patients, and they're trained to deal with their psyches. Physicians should be trained to encourage that same sensitivity.

"We need to pay more attention to the stress that the students have to deal with. The problem of uncertainty, of dealing with failures and mistakes, and the fear that you don't know the answers. We need to work with students, to help them express their feelings and learn to understand themselves and what they're going through. Medical students and doctors don't usually know how to ask for help. There can be a lot of emotional suffering in training, a lot of inner conflict, and they feel they have to hide and suppress it. They would make better doctors if they knew how to deal with their feelings.

"I almost dropped out of my residency. I had one month where five patients died, and I didn't know how to cope with it. I felt I was a failure because my job was to save them and I couldn't. I think it's important that these kinds of issues are talked about, to prepare doctors for what they're going to deal with in a more realistic way.

"If you care about patients, you're going to feel some pain when they suffer or die. The solution is usually to develop a certain detachment, but we can't let that affect how we *treat* people. We can't do that at the expense of caring. It's hard, but we have to teach people to be vigilant about what they're feeling. That kind of introspection and psychological acumen ought to be part of our training, but no one pays any attention to the psyche and the soul of future doctors. We should make sure that medical students have time to think about who they are and why they're there."

TOWARD A NEW FLEXNER REPORT

Reforming training procedures will not, by itself, solve the many institutional problems facing medicine today. Questions of cost, insurance, regulation, access to resources, and the like involve social, economic, and political forces beyond the scope of our respondents' remarks. However, many of our doctors believed that the future of medicine depends as much on the sphere of private practice as on public policy. The quality of medical care, they felt, is reflected first and foremost in the fundamental dyad of the physician-patient relationship.

In that context, two of our doctors ventured detailed predictions that seemed particularly insightful, if not prescient. First, a G.P. in Los Angeles: "Medicine in the twenty-first century will surpass our wildest futuristic visions, but it will also be very old-fashioned. Two people talking about this subject in the year 2040 will say we were totally primitive in treating cancer by hacking pieces out of people. They'll be using natural substances to mobilize the body's own forces to destroy aberrant cells. They'll think we were barbarians for performing surgery willy-nilly and ingesting chemicals with awful side effects. They'll think it absurd that we thought we were waging war against disease at the same time we were making the whole planet an un-healthy environment.

"In the future, prevention will be on equal footing with treatment. We will take it for granted that the mind and emotions influence the course of disease. Remedies will be manufactured with more concern for side effects and taken more directly from the natural world of plants and minerals. The influence of environmental toxins will be better understood, and public policy will be more supportive of those concerns. Primary physicians will be trained to know their patients intimately and observe the verities of comfort, concern, and compassion. In that respect, the future will be more like the past, when the traditional country doctor, or the neighborhood doctor, knew his patients and their families intimately and was cognizant of their health needs."

The other would-be prophet was a New York internist who spoke of the need for a more integrated health-care system: "The U.S. lacks an overall design that takes full advantage of what we know about disease and can mobilize all the appropriate persons and organizations when an individual gets sick. I hope in the future that the family doctor will be like a home room teacher, someone who coordinates all the resources necessary to manage your condition, whether you need a specialist, a technician, an acupuncturist, a psychotherapist, a career counselor, a support group, child care, social worker, or whatever. So many things affect our health and so many services are relevant, but as it is now, it's an ad hoc system. You enter it haphazardly, and it can be chaotic, redundant, and inefficient. We need to find an orderly way for people to enter the system at the level appropriate to their need.

"This is a tragedy. For one thing, a lot of the patients' needs fail to be met because no one has the whole picture in mind. For another, it costs society a lot of money because if a patient doesn't get what he needs in the early stages, he keeps getting sick, and maybe ends up needing expensive tests or surgery that could have been avoided.

"We need to find a way to integrate the system. It's not going to be easy, with all the different interest groups, lobbyists, bureaucrats, and jurisdictional hassles, but, on the other hand, it's not a blue sky proposition. We already have most of the elements in place. It's a question of coordination and proper allocation, of bringing the elements together in the proper way, so we can better implement the capabilities we now have. You can see glimpses of a coordinated system in Canada and England and even parts of the Third World.

"For example, when I was in Nicaragua, I saw a desperately poor country with hardly any resources, but yet it was still able to develop a highly useful system. They have field offices in every village of a certain size, and in each one there is a doctor, nurse, and a mental health counselor. These little units are scattered throughout the countryside, and they don't deal exclusively with physical illnesses. They deal with the patient's family, employment, and other situations that relate to their health. If a specialist is needed, the patient is taken to one in the nearest city. Their equipment and knowledge are primitive compared to ours, but there's an admirable attempt to coordinate what they have. Imagine what we could do if we integrated our resources more systematically."

Surely, the future will see new miracle cures, and wondrous technologies will conquer killer diseases and continue to extend the average life span. But, that same heroic trend may further exacerbate certain problems, such as unrealistic expectations, increased costs, greater specialization, and the impersonal atmosphere decried by many of the physicians we interviewed. Perhaps the suggestions of our respondents—e.g., to enhance the psychological fitness and sensitivity of doctors, to provide more personal attention to patients, and to encourage greater latitude and creativity in selecting treatments—will assert a balancing influence on the future practice of medicine.

In that regard, it is interesting to recall that early in this century, when medicine was at a crossroads marked by confusion and chaos, the Flexner Report, like the doctors in our survey, focused its call for reform on medical training. Perhaps the times demand a contemporary equivalent of the Flexner Report: a coherent, well-researched delineation of the state of medicine and a mandate for a new direction. Given the complexity of today's circumstances, this is no simple task, but one hopes that an appropriate body will take up the challenge. One also hopes that a modern version of the Flexner Report will be as inclusive as its predecessor was exclusionary; that it will recognize the important role that social, environmental and psychological factors play in the disease process; that it can provide a unifying theoretical framework for medicine into the next century; that its focal point will be the needs of patients, and its recommendations for the training of physicians will focus on how to best fulfill those needs.

In the meantime, it is important for all of us to realize that the future of medicine is, to some extent, in our hands. We are well advised to assume responsibility for our own health and to approach the medical marketplace as wise consumers. This requires taking an active role in making decisions and educating ourselves about the full range of health matters, including economic, legislative and political issues concerning health care. At the same time, we should increase our awareness of our bodies and various symptoms that arise. We should ask ourselves what we want from our relationships with our doctors and communicate clearly with them. We should not assume our doctors know everything, or even that they know best, and we should not be afraid of wasting their time or sounding foolish by asking questions. While we are each only one patient among millions, we can nevertheless make a major contribution to the future of health care by insisting on the best possible treatment and the most comprehensive information, understanding our own bodies, and establishing a co-operative and meaningful partnership with our doctors.

FINDING AND WORKING WITH AN ALTERNATIVE PHYSICIAN

When we completed this book, it occurred to us that readers might seek out some of the unconventional treatments described, or find themselves in an examining room with a doctor who recommends them. What follows are suggestions and caveats to help guide your choices regarding alternative medicine:

1. *Start with a medical doctor.* In large urban areas, you can find non-physician practitioners for virtually every form of alternative treatment. Many are well trained and adept at administering acupuncture, dispensing homeopathic or herbal remedies, teaching yoga or meditation, prescribing nutritional supplements, and so on. But, with rare exceptions, these lay specialists can't match the training of medical doctors or their comprehensive repertoire of diagnostic procedures. M.D.s can also combine alternative and mainstream procedures as needed, whereas lay practitioners are limited to their specialties.

It should be noted, however, that a physician who studied an alternative procedure informally might actually have less experience and skill than a lay specialist. In some cases, the licensing and certification requirements for unconventional healers are quite stringent; yet, M.D.s may not be required to meet those additional standards.

Nevertheless, you are well advised to see a medical doctor as your point of entry. If the physician is not trained in the alternative treatment you're interested in, he might direct you to a colleague or a lay practitioner, just as he might recommend a psychiatrist or a physical therapist. By beginning with a physician, you will at least be assured of a presumptive diagnosis and a responsible referral. Ideally, your physician can serve as a head coach who monitors and oversees the other members of your medical team.

2. *Get a recommendation you can trust.* If you are looking for a physician who employs alternative practices, the best place to begin is with friends and family members. In addition, you might inquire at local hospitals, clinics, and medical schools, or unusual sources such as health food markets and phone directories where holistic clinics and individual practitioners might be listed. Also, the reference sections of most local libraries contain various directories and rosters of professional organizations such as the American Osteopathic Association and *The North American Holistic Resources Directory.* Your state and local societies for naturopaths and chiropractors may also assist you, or you might contact the National Committee for the Certification of Acupuncturists at 1424 16th St., N.W.; Washington, D.C. 20036, or the National Center of Homeopathy at 1500 Massachusetts Ave., N.W.; Washington, D.C. 20005.

3. *Don't hesitate to ask questions.* If your doctor recommends an unusual procedure, treat it the same way you would any medical recommendation: ask every question that comes to mind. Exactly why is it recommended? What results can you expect? Are there potential side effects?

Once you are adequately informed, you can make an educated choice as to whether the treatment is something you care to try. If you don't feel comfortable with either the remedy or the individual practitioner, you are well advised to look elsewhere.

4. *Beware of fanatics.* In medicine, as in all professions, fads come and go. Just as some doctors are closed-minded when it comes to new

and different treatments, others can be overzealous. Warning flags should go up if a doctor seems to make excessive claims for a particular procedure or prescribes it without benefit of a thorough diagnostic workup. Be especially wary of those who are overtly hostile to mainstream medicine or ridicule standard procedures.

5. *Question your own motives.* Are you drawn to the procedure because you are desperate to believe in something? It's easy to get excited about something new and different, especially if it resonates with your hopes for a complete and painless cure. Some alternative treatments require more involvement from the patient. Are you willing to make the effort and give the procedure a proper chance to work?

7. *Do you trust the physician?* Agreeing to a treatment plan, whether mainstream or alternative, involves some degree of faith. Consider the personal chemistry between you and the doctor. Is he responsive to you? Does he listen to your concerns and understand your priorities? Does he take the time to answer your questions, explain his procedures, and assuage your fears? Is he genuinely concerned for your welfare?

In the final analysis, you can do no better than to hold your doctor to these simple standards from the Hippocratic Oath, which was written more than two thousand years ago and is still recited by graduating physicians today: "I will follow that system of regimen which, according to my ability and judgment, I consider for the benefit of my patients, and abstain from whatever is deleterious and mischievous."

INDEX

One of the purposes for writing *A Different Kind of Healing* was to provide physicians with the opportunity to share thought-provoking observations and their experiences with unusual treatments. We now hope to provide a forum for the exchange of additional information along these lines and to establish a data base for future research and hypothesis building. We invite accounts of your personal observations and experiences. Please send them to A Different Kind of Healing, 138 Ocean Way, Santa Monica, CA 90402. Both signed and anonymous contributions are welcome.

ABOUT THE AUTHORS

Oscar Janiger, M.D., has been a practicing psychiatrist and university professor for more than forty years. Formerly the Co-director of Residency Training at Metropolitan State Hospital in Norwalk, California, and Research Director of the Holmes Center for Research in Holistic Healing, he is currently Associate Clinical Professor in the

Department of Psychiatry and Human Behavior, University of California at Irvine. He lives in Santa Monica, California.

Philip Goldberg is the author or coauthor of eleven nonfiction books, including *The Intuitive Edge, Executive Health,* and the forthcoming *How to Stay Sane in a Crazy World.* A full-time writer, he also writes fiction and screenplays. His novel *This Is Next Year* is currently in development as a feature film. Born and raised in New York, he now lives in Los Angeles.

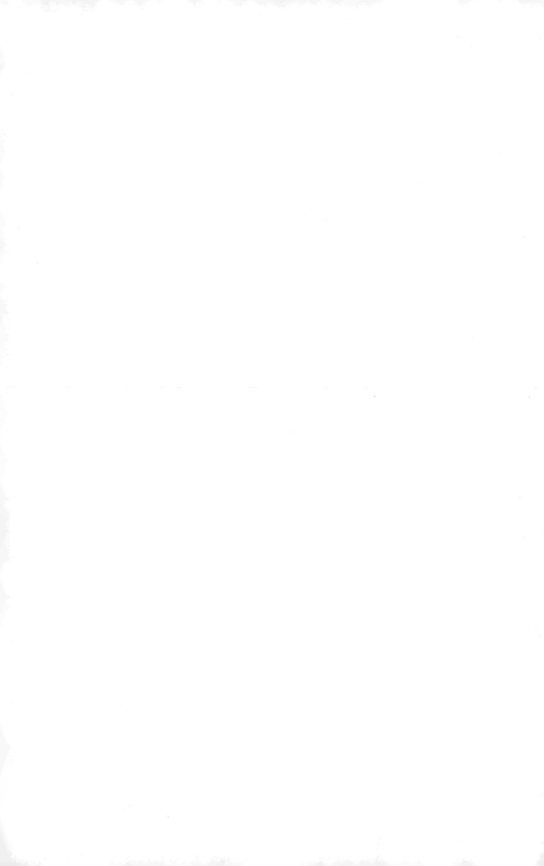